Carmen Roman

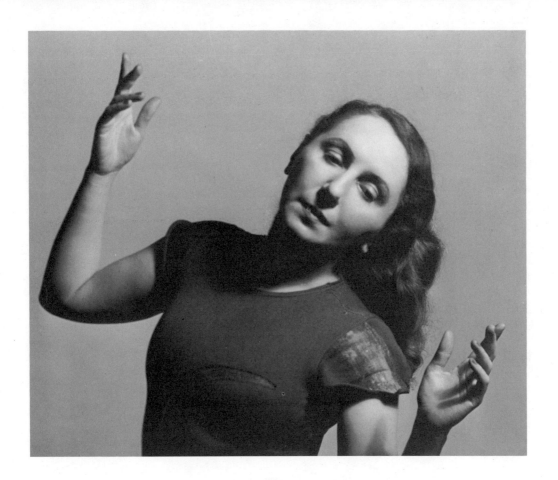

Collected Works by and about

BLANCHE EVAN
Unedited

DANCER, TEACHER, WRITER
DANCE/MOVEMENT/WORD THERAPIST

January 28, 1909 — December 24, 1982

Compiled by Ruth Gordon Benov

Copyright 1991

Blanche Evan Dance Foundation

Dedicated

To

The memory of <u>Blanche Evan</u> who helped so many to unify mind, body and spirit through her teaching of creative dance and her dance/movement/word therapy.

The contents of this book have been compiled by:

Ruth Gordon Benov

with assistance from

Bonnie Bernstein

Anne Krantz

Barbara Melson

Iris Rifkin-Gainer

TABLE OF CONTENTS

Material has been reprinted with permission and sources are indicated.

PREFACE

Because of the growing interest in the work of Blanche Evan and frequent inquiries about sources for her writings, it was felt that a publication of her collected works would be utile. Thus this book came to be.

This collection represents all published works about and by Ms. Evan. Regretfully, her unpublished works could not be included here. However, a listing of these works is provided.

The material is organized chronologically to show the growth of the person and the social, artistic and political climate in which artists of that time struggled and grew.

In order to be as faithful as possible to the original documents, no changes or corrections were made in spelling, punctuation or typographical inconsistencies.

This work is a tribute to Blanche Evan the dancer, the writer, the therapist.

--Ruth Gordon Benov

Homage to My Aunt
Read by Carol Evan McKeand
at services, N.Y.C., December 28, 1982

BLANCHE EVAN
In Memory
December 24th, 1982

Meeting: robust laughs still fresh.

Going: tears surge.

Departing feast already heart-smiting.

Dreary city, among other things, brings sorrow.

Sky biting cold, distant mountains clean.

Sun at dusk; long river rushes.

Weigh anchor.   You recede into the distance.

And at the prow you still stand.

Seeing Tsu-san Off at Ch'i-chou

Wang Wei (701-761 A.D.)

Homage to Our Teacher

By Bonnie Bernstein, Anne Krantz,
Barbara Melson, Iris Rifkin-Gainer

Read by Barbara Melson at services, New York City December 28, 1982

Blanche Evan, pioneer in the fields of dance, choreography, dance teaching and dance therapy for the neurotic client, died December 24, 1982 in New York City.

Her absolute belief in the power of dance and her view of the individual's basic potential for growth and change are among the qualities which made her an inspiring and ever-evolving dance therapist who profoundly touched the lives of many.

Miss Evan had her own studio in New York City from 1934 to 1975, and founded the Dance Therapy Centre, the first nucleus of Dance Therapy for the normal neurotic urban adult, in 1967. She had presented her material at Universities and in workshops throughout the United States and was scheduled to travel to the West Coast to teach at the time of her death.

As a young dancer, Miss Evan studied with Bird Larson. Later she trained at the Adler Institute of Individual Psychology. Her publications "The Child's World: Its Relation to Dance Pedagogy" and "Packet of Pieces: Dance Therapy for the Neurotic Client" as well as films made between 1935 and 1977 are filed in the Lincoln Center Archives. Miss Evan was a founding member of the A.D.T.A. and was honored by the organization at the October 1982 Conference.

Miss Evan has stated "my objective...is the integration of dance _with_ therapy, so that it becomes one...'Dance: A Basic Therapy.'"

Her personal and professional contribution is immeasurable. She will be deeply missed.

VITAE

Blanche Evan began her own studio/school in 1934.

Her Principal Teachers:

Fundamental training in creative dance with Bird Larson

Supplemental training in the work of Mary Wigman, Martha Graham, Harald Kreutzberg and Hanya Holm

Cecchetti Ballet with Ella Daganova

Ballet with Vilzak-Shollar-Tarasoff

Choreography with Louis Horst and Doris Humphrey

Mensendieck work in body mechanics

Dalcroze Eurhythmics

Ethnic and Spanish Dance with La Meri and Veola

Films:

Two Films on Blanche Evan's work in therapy and one on basics of her system on Functional Technique are in the permanent film archives of the Dance Collection at Lincoln Center, New York City.

As performer - From beginning to the end of her life:

Performed in solo and joint recitals:

Benjamin Franklin High School, Norwalk, Conn.

City College of New York City

Dance Guild at Vanderbilt Theatre, New York City and Newark, N.J.

Provincetown Players' Production of "Orpheus", Mass.

Elizabeth Peabody Playhouse, Boston, Mass.

Elizabeth Peabody Theatre, Boston, Mass.

Garrison Playhouse, New York City

Hecksher Theatre, New York City

Humphrey-Weidman Studio, New York City

Hunter College, New York City

Master Institute Theatre, New York City

Max Reinhardt's production "Eternal Road," New York City

Moscow, Leningrad, U.S.S.R.

New School for Social Research, New York City

New York Labor Stage Theatre, New York City

North Carolina College for Negroes, Durham, N.C.

Roerich Hall, New York City

St. James Theatre, New York City

Shaw University, Raleigh, N.C.

Studio Theatre, New York City

Town Hall, New York City

Victoria Hall and His Majesty's Theatre, Montreal

Wheeling Symphony Orchestra, Wheeling, W.Va.

Lecturer/Teacher - From beginning to the end of her life:

A.D.T.A. Workshop, New York City

Alfred Adler Institute, Adjunctive Therapist, New York City

Albertina Rasch, New York City

American Dance Association, New York City

Bellevue Childrens Psychiatric Ward, New York City

Benjamin Franklin High School, Norwalk, Conn.

Boulder, Colo.

Carnegie Recital Hall, New York City

Dance Guild, New York City

Denver, Colo.

Educational Alliance, New York City

Hunter College, New York City

McGill University, Canada

Neighborhood Music School Research, New York City

New School for Social Research, New York City

New York University, New York City

North Carolina College, Durham, N.C.

Rebell Arts, New York City

Roerich Museum, New York City

San Francisco, Calif.

Sedona, Ariz.

Settlement House, New York City

Shaw University, Raleigh, N.C.

Studio Caravan, New York City

Studio Theatre, New York City

YWCA, Stamford Conn.

*As Dance Movement/Word Therapist, in her latter years she devoted all of her time to her private practice and group workshops.

She was invited to conduct sessions in her therapy method to graduate dance therapy programs at colleges in the United States.

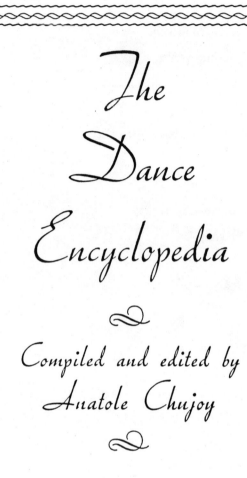

The

Dance

Encyclopedia

Compiled and edited by

Anatole Chujoy

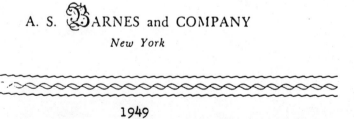

A. S. BARNES and COMPANY

New York

1949

Evan, Blanche, contemporary dancer and teacher; b. New York City; studied with *Bird Larson, Hanya Holm, Martha Graham, Ella Dagnova, Harald Kreutzberg, Doris Humphrey, Dalcroze, Vilzak-Shollar, La Meri,* Veola. Has appeared in solo and joint recitals in various N.Y. theatres; in Norwalk, Conn.; Newark, N.J.; Boston, Mass.; Moscow, U.S.S.R. (1935-37). Choreographs own dances. Has taught, lectured and given demonstrations in various schools and colleges since 1933; contributed to Theatre Arts, *Dance Magazine,* Parent's Magazine, Jewish, Survey, etc. Has had own studio in N.Y. since 1934.

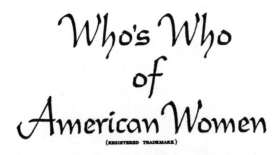

Who's Who of American Women
(REGISTERED TRADEMARK)

A BIOGRAPHICAL DICTIONARY OF
NOTABLE LIVING AMERICAN WOMEN

THIRD EDITION

(1964-1965)

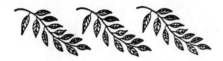

INCORPORATED—A NON-PROFIT
FOUNDATION
(The A. N. Marquis Company—Founded 1897)
Marquis Publications Building
210 EAST OHIO STREET
CHICAGO-11 USA

311

Evan, Blanche Evelyn, dancer; b. N.Y.C., Jan. 28, 1909; d. Julius and Anna (Ivan) Chermerinsky; pvt. study dancing, 1918-46; student Hunter Coll., 1927-30; m. Lionel Hillel Berman, July 7, 1936 (div. Apr.1947). Soloist, group recitals in N.Y., Conn., N.J., Mass., Can., W.Va., USSR, 1927-47; owner, operator Sch. Creative Dance, N.Y.C., 1934--; mem. cast Max Reinhardt's Eternal Road, N.Y.C., 1936-37. Creator Film Studies of Dance, 1936; dance therapist, 1951--; faculty mem. Master Inst., N.Y.C., 1933-34, Albertina Rasch, 1933-35, Neighborhood Music Sch., 1942-44, settlement houses, 1933-40; dance therapist Bellevue Children's Psychiat. Ward, N.Y.C. 1943; spl. summer faculty N.C. Coll. for Negroes, 1947; co-chmn. adjunctive therapies com. Alfred Adler Inst. Individual Psychology, 1959. Mem Am. Dance Assn. (exec. pres. dance guild and chmn. forums com. 1935-37). Contbr. numerous articles on dance theory, pedagogy, therapy to dance and popular mags., 1935-59. Office: 133 2d Av., N.Y.C. 3.

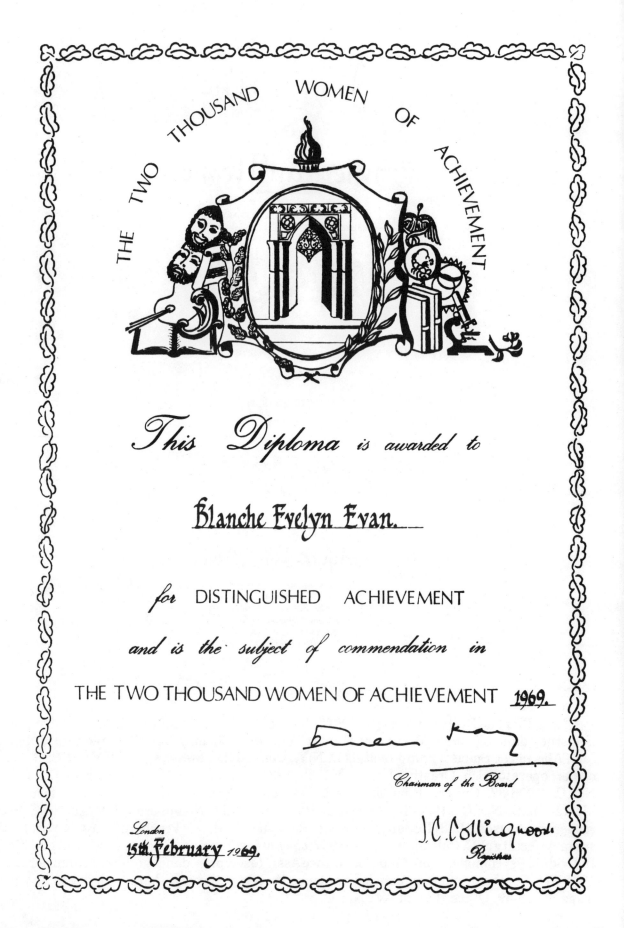

THE TWO THOUSAND WOMEN OF ACHIEVEMENT

This Diploma is awarded to

Blanche Evelyn Evan.

for DISTINGUISHED ACHIEVEMENT

and is the subject of commendation in

THE TWO THOUSAND WOMEN OF ACHIEVEMENT 1969.

Chairman of the Board

J. C. Collingwood.
Registrar

London
15th February 1969.

The Dance Therapy Centre
Blanche Evan, Director

5 West 20 Street
New York, N.Y. 10011
UN5-6505

In 1967, Blanche Evan established the Dance Therapy Centre. The following statements are excerpts from the brochures:

In the BLANCHE EVAN SCHOOL, technique is not treated as an amputated limb of Dance, but rather as one of its functional organs. It is presented so that its pursuit does not become a block to creative spontaneity...The work does not negate form but seeks a new form that is the result of a union of unmannered technique with the creative use of content.

Each participant in Creative dance is guided to know her own body's gamut of movement and to make it the instrument for expressing emotions. Dance thus fulfills the need of a psycho-physical union.

THE DANCE THERAPY CENTRE the first in New York, will open its doors to the public on September 17, 1967. It is the dream-come-true of Blanche Evan who will direct its activities and staff it with trainees who have completed the courses created by Miss Evan in Dance Therapy. Guest lecturers and teachers will be invited at times.

Bi-monthly forums and introductory classes will be open to the public. Members of the Centre will enjoy the reference use of the Dance library and vast music collection of Blanche Evan, at specified hours at the Centre.

The main spine of the Centre will consist of Dance classes for adults oriented to Dance therapy, and to group and private sessions of Dance therapy.

The Centre is an extension of the Dance therapy work carried on for the past ten years at the Blanche Evan School of Creative Dance and Therapy.

WHY A DANCE THERAPY CENTRE? It will provide:

a place for those seeking better health through body movement and Dance

a place for the public to learn about the advantages and accessibility of Dance Therapy

a place where doctors, psychotherapists, social workers, counselors, and other workers in mental health can ask questions about Dance Therapy as an adjunct for their clients

a place where PERFORMING ARTISTS, ACTORS, MUSICIANS, DANCERS, can find release of tension and where they can broaden their use of the body as an unblocked medium of expression

a place where STUDENTS AND MEMBERS can meet at informal forums; and can read about Dance, and can listen to music-for-dance

a place where WELCOME will be extended to the disabled, and to the retarded child, for Dance therapy a place where the adult who wants to relax, to move and to dance, to realign posture, to confront the body image, and to express the self, can be assured of:

a. functional body movement and non-mannered technique

b. the experience of uncluttered and depth improvisation

and a place where, in classes, the INDIVIDUAL STUDENT is treated AS and individual

STAFF

The school and Centre are staffed only by adults trained by Blanche Evan over a period of years.

For 1967: Toni Lacativa, Macia Halkin, Iris Rifkin, Nancy Spanier (on leave), Guest Teacher for Afro work — Howard Halyard

Teacher for children with learning dysfunction, sense deprivation, retardation — Ruth G. Benov

The Published Works

of

Blanche Evan

1934 — 1982

April, 1934   Price 10 cents

New Theatre

DRAMA • FILM • DANCE

The Dance
AN OPEN LETTER
To Workers' Dance Groups

The Revolutionary Dance movement is without question vital and important, and there is every reason to believe that it will eventually assert itself in the non-political field of dance activity in America. The recent dance program given at City College, at which all the revolutionary dance groups in and near New York appeared, has brought several issues to the fore, which I, as representative of many politically sympathetic, professional dancers, would like to have discussed.

What is the aim of the proletarian dance? Is it to proselytize? Does it wish to state the problems of the proletariat, or solve them as well? Is it to renew the enthusiasm of convinced class-conscious people? Is it to afford a method of entertainment to them that will yet be within the realm of their deepest convictions? Does it wish to create an art form that has a single and definite ideology, or does it wish to establish a form of propaganda that uses *the dance as its medium?* Of course, there is no reason to limit the proletarian dance to any one of these objectives; but it seems to me that when composing a revolutionary dance, one of the first considerations should be its ultimate purpose, since that purpose must mould the form of the dance.

If a dance attempts to convert, it must try to reach an audience outside its own circle. Accordingly, the political issue must be kept in the background, and the dance must carry its message by a more emotional ideology. By doing this, a place is made immediately on programs that would not consent to the appearance of such dances, were the political statement made too obtrusive. Might it not be advantageous to form an "Innocents" dance organization that would create within the workers' ideology, but that would direct its efforts to reaching outside audiences?

The Joos interview of the New Theater ended with a regret that Joos had stated his problem, but had offered no solution. In America, we are still lacking awareness of these problems. Might it not be of value to spend energy in presenting the worker's difficulties as such, as often and to as many different audiences as possible? It is done in literature; why not in dance? It is obvious that had Joos ended his "Green Table" in formal propaganda fashion, he would never have been permitted to play on Broadway at all, and thousands of people would have been denied witnessing this effective statement of the horrors of war.

From the viewpoint of the pure, political propagandist, the criticism of the ending of the "Green Table" is open to question. No one can deny the importance of the dramatic in any propaganda work. Could a final scene shooting down the politicians, even figuratively, have been more effective than the biting satire, the contrast of the preceding scenes of the effects of war with unconcerned-ness of the Green Table diplomats? Granted that there is but one solution to the workers' problem, does it not rather weaken than strengthen every dance, by ending it with the symbolic singing of the Internationale? The audience might be carried away by the dramatic mistreatment of the Negro in the dance called "Southern Holiday"; and psychologically, it might be much more effective to leave him mistreated, than to see his problem solved so easily by the onrush of red-coated dancers.

Our third question leads us back to the City College performance. Why did the Duncan Group, which despite its somewhat technical immaturity, and lack of that sophistication which, for instance, the Theatre Union Groups possessed receive the biggest ovation of the evening? Was it despite these reasons, or because of them? Technical immaturity is nothing to boast of but simplicity of form and directness of statement seem best suited for said purpose. Was it not also, because on a program of woe and struggle, it gave the proletarian an idea of the joy that might await him in the future? This is not pure entertainment. It is propaganda of a different sort. It lifts the worker for the moment into a better and freer world that is still very much his own world. The worker needs relaxation. The dance seems, of all arts, best suited to give it to him.

Apparently, the policy of the groups is divided: to create dances that find their inspiration in the problems of the worker, or to create propaganda that uses the dance as its medium. In the latter case, the dancers still commit themselves to follow a certain procedure, and to recognize the limitations implied in the activity of "the dance." It is platitudinous to say that the dance is movement of the body; that what then is expressed, is done so, and is projected through body movement.

This is not the purist speaking. One usually finds that remaining within the medium produces a better result than going outside it. The surrealist movement in painting, in which painters pasted on their canvases everything from glass to orange skins, had a short life; whereas, the true innovators, who discovered different means of using paints and brushes, have had a lasting significance. The revolutionary dancer, if she wishes to broaden the possibilities of expression in her medium, can do a great deal in broadening the possibilities of movement within the body, and within space, by means of theatrical use of platforms, levels, etc.

An idea in itself, may be a very powerful one; but if it is not an idea that can express itself in movement, if it is not a dance idea, or rather a danceable idea, it does not belong in dance propaganda, but might be more effective in literary, pantomimic, or spoken form. An idea like "The Blue Eagle," one of the New Dance Group's offerings, is first of all a broad *topic*, an intellectual idea, involving numerous problems of politics, economy, nationalism, internationalism. It has within it *many* motives for the legitimate theatre or for the agitprop groups. The N. R. A. signs, carried by two of the dancers, in helping to fortify the intellectual concept, minimized even the possibility of regarding the idea of N. R. A. as symbolic—if that's what the group wished its audience to do.

The dance propagandists might succeed in creating more effective and more inspiring dances if they held more consideration for the medium which they have chosen to employ.

—Blanche Evan

NEW

OCTOBER, 1934

THEATRE

10¢

THE STAR SPANGLED DANCE

By Blanche Evan

The chauvinistic trend of the modern dance in this country burst forth with unmistakable clarity of intent this year. Down with foreign methods, foreign dance art, foreign-born dancers. Let themes, manner, music, even dance musicians be American. Just how many generations back the dancer's American ancestry must extend, has not been formulated—yet! (How many does Hitler ordain to qualify as a pure Aryan?)

The national dance movement has chosen as its spokesman the only so-called modern dance publication in America, the *Dance Observer*; "so-called" because this magazine makes plain its intention of supporting not the modern dance, but only the American manifestation of the modern dance. From cover to cover, the contents refer to the American dance, American theme, American manner, American music. It is even lamented that American modern dance can't "buy American". In its anxiety to relate the work of the American modern dancer to America, we stumble across the most fantastic relationships.

For instance, in speaking of American theme, we read that the "oldest and most colorful strains in American life have been the most attractive as material—the Negro, the Indian, and the Jew!" And speaking of Jewish life in America, we are given a long list of Chassidic, Palestinian, and racial references, that have as much to do with America as the festival ceremonies of the Tibetan Lamas. Must the American dancer force the legitimacy of the "American" theme to this extent? Must she pick up a book on Indian lore, on Negro spirituals, or on Jewish religious rites if she is to dance America? The only relationship that an American dancer can truthfully establish between herself and these most "colorful" strains, lies, perhaps in this: that her ancestors robbed the Indians of their land, the Negroes continue to be enslaved on the pretext of racial inferiority, and the Jews are still subjected to anti-semitism.

But such an interpretation of America would be far from acceptable. The same article, referred to above, states very definitely that not only shall we dance the American theme, but also that we shall find our best material in the dead and forgotten past.

"Oddly enough," it continues, "all three (the Negro, Indian, and Jew) are only interesting when they act least in accordance with their times and surroundings. We visualize the Negro—open-mouthed, spread-fingered, feet shuffling to the spiritual he is singing; the Indian—rattle in one hand, pine-branch in the other, stamping in a breath-taking rhythm that unites him with the earth and elements; the Jew —flowing white beard, a prayer shawl and phylacteries, swaying while he intones his prayers. All three are still existent, yet already belong to the past. This is an ideal combination for the seeker of material for he can study the material when it is no longer agitated by the present." Back to the tranquil past! Back to the American revolution, the War of 1812, the Civil War, the War of 1898, the World War!

Who are our representative "American-born" dancers? What have they danced about? Two of the latest programs of Humphrey-Weidman, and Graham, yield the titles: "Alcina Suite", Dionysiaques",

"Exhibition Piece", "Dithyrambic". "Ekstasis", "Primitive Mysteries...Hymn to the Virgin", etc. What, in their programs reveals America? But wait. We are told that "the manner more than the material would have to be relied upon to be American." What is happening to the ideal of the modern dance? To its prime motive of individuality? Why did it ever bother to revolt against the academicism of the ballet, if it is to be dragged back again into formulae of manner and mannerism?

Let us burst the last bubble of the national-dance war-cry, the native dancer, "American-born". Let us remember for purposes of clarification—and beautiful burlesque—that Picasso, the most typical of the modern French school in painting, was a *Spanish Jew!* Let us remember for purposes of safety, that the modern dance world is limited enough, and that confining it to the American-born would just about wipe it out of existence altogether.

What is left of the American this-and-that in the modern dance? It is obvious that the desire to be American and to express America is being used as a pretext to promote the idea of chauvinistic art--and for no other purpose. Since the modern dance has had its only significant development in America and Germany, the insinuation is unmistakable: "Down with German methods, German dance art, artists, teachers."

Even the most American of American dancers or critics cannot deny that the pure modern dance in Germany had reached great heights of development while the "modern" dancers in America were still toying with bracelets in Oriental impressions. The new dance left homeless by Isadora's death, was picked up in Germany--not in America. Laban wove the cloth--and Wigman cut the pattern. But Laban and Wigman did not concentrate on their own national German characteristics; they went about with all the scientific and artistic fervor they could command, to clarify and to develop a universal basis for the modern dance. And they did. The Wigman pedagogy remains one of the few we have in America today that attempts to drive to the universal roots of the modern dance, and not to encrust these roots with personal or national interpretations.

Nationalism and art are as incongruous as nationalism and science. The researches of Laban, the artistry of Wigman, the pedagogy of the Wigman method are not German, any more than the theories of Einstein are. The dance, because its body movement is a science and its expression an art, is universal. Accordingly the theoretical problems and their solution are also universal. The modern dance is not rooted in any soil. Its exponents in America are struggling with the same problems as those in Germany or in England: problems of space and time, composition, accompaniment, pedagogy, notation. These are problems that are fundamental to the art, and not indigenous to any geographical area.

It seems extremely probable that in a peaceful, unruffled epoch, an artist would be quite susceptible to both the local and the national color of life. Living in the Rockies of America, theme and manner would naturally not be the same as if he lived in a big industrial city; and they would certainly take on a different character if he went to live in and absorb the life of a foreign country--as the Frenchman Gaugin proved in his Tahitian venture. But in a world so filled with action, where life is not localized, but transmits itself through every vein of existence, not only does the local color lose itself in the national, but the national loses itself in the international, and that, in turn, in the universal. There are rhythms vibrating through the world which a sensitive artist cannot escape; the rhythms of a stark reality, of strife, conflict, change, of submission to destruction, or of the renewal of energy in the search for a better world. The rhythm travels to the far corners of the earth--its waves encompass the artists not only within an art, but within all the arts, and unite them in one powerful surge.

Let American modern dancers rid themselves of their escape in the past. Let them cease to seek and to study that "material...no longer agitated by the present." Let them abandon their "patriotic" isolation. Let them open their beings to the strength of the world rhythm. In the spirit of all true workers, let them take their German co-dancers by the hand, and strive together toward the fertile realm of the modern dance.

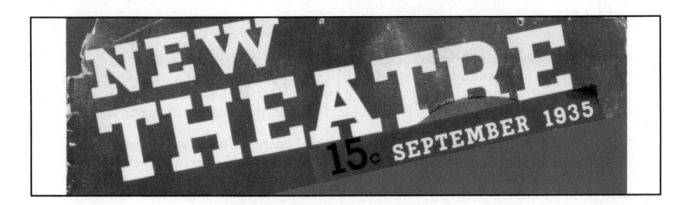

NEW THEATRE

15c SEPTEMBER 1935

The Fokine Ballets
By BLANCHE EVAN

I went eagerly to the Stadium this summer in search of the "miracle" of choreography of which John Martin spoke in his review of *Scheherazade*. During the progress of the performance my eagerness was very quickly transformed into disappointment. The "tired business man" has as his weekly fare, in almost any movie house presentation, this kind of pseudo-choreographic miracle. The handling of ensemble was weak in comparison with any one of the Joos ballets, and painfully weak in comparison with the least interesting of Humphrey's or Graham's group compositions. How monotonous the repeated use of cliche poses--Maxfield Parrish equally in evidence in the Oriental setting of *Scheherazade* and in what the program notes termed "pure dancing," the presentation *Elves*.

It is true that ballets like *Scheherazade*, created in 1910, were considered extremely radical from the point of view of dance form. It is true they were of immense importance in the development of the art of the dance and as a vehicle for the best musicians and stage designers of the time. But that is no reason why they in themselves could not have been integral pieces of choreographic form able to stand the test of revival. By analogy, the paintings of Picasso and Braque who also were the insurgents of their time have already become classic. Again one must disagree with John Martin when he says that only the passage of time will give these ballets "sufficient mellowness of perspective to assume a place in any permanent repertoire." Ballets like *Scheherazade* do not hold within them a single germ to make them worthy of resurrection as great works of choreographic art in the present or in the future.

The reason for this consummate failure of so widely heralded a ballet as *Scheherazade* embraces the historical, technical, and social phases of ballet in general.

The Degeneracy of Ballet--The Perugini definition of the art of ballet is "a series of solo and concerted dances with mimetic actions, accompanied by music and scenic accessories telling a story." Any balletomane in the world will tell you that without the complete harmony of all these elements, a ballet performance must be a failure. The ballet school which is the nucleus of ballet theatre production has followed in America a direct line of degeneracy. The Russian ballet masters who emigrated to America forced ballet into this degeneracy by commercializing their schools, by eliminating all study of the expressive medium of the ballet, which is pantomime, by allowing mere children to work in toe slippers before any muscular development had taken place, and finally by emasculating the artistic forces of ballet until only the skeleton of technique was left. Without the combination of great pantomimic artistry with technical skill, the art of ballet cannot exist. The performance of Fokine's pupils at the Stadium proved this. Even if Fokine's choreography for *Scheherazade* were great, his dancers who to-day are prepared to execute only the correct *number* of steps (and this is being generous to the cast) cheapen and vulgarize the work by their utter ignorance of mime and by their complete lack of sensitive interpretation. The love scenes of Zobeide, the heroine of *Scheherazade*, executed in the manner of the Folies Bergeres, are a good example. The same choreography handled by Karsavina and Nijinsky must certainly have shone to better advantage. Stripped of the assistance of great expressive artists, the Fokine choreography does not stand as exciting, pure formal design. It becomes in this case decidedly barren and banal.

Motivation in Creation--It is not *chiefly* that there is "unemployment and social upheaval" today, as John Martin says, that we cannot be "seriously carried away" by the revival of *Scheherazade*. It is rather that at the time of its creation, in 1910, the motivation for creation had no attachment to reality. Not only was it detached from the contemporary scene. Fokine did not even *interpret* the atmosphere in which it was placed, but merely presented a conventional viewpoint in a stereotyped setting. Isadora Duncan also went to a foreign source for her material. But in her case, she strove to capture the spirit of the Greeks, rather than merely to reproduce a Greek scene.

Sunk in the subsidies of the Imperial Court of Russia and in the capitalists' court that followed Diaghileff, Fokine believed be could shut his eyes to the burning realities of the world in which he lived. In 1910, there were the same preparation for war as there are today; the same savage persecution of racial and religious minorities as occurs in Hitler Germany. Five years before, the Russian masses returning from the Russo-Japanese War had fought a bloody civil war. Unlike the great Russian writers of the same period, such as Gorki, Fokine worked with themes arbitrarily and depended for their vitality on the gorgeous decor of Bakst in which they were dressed.

There was nothing real in the motivation and nothing enduring in the results.

Ballet *can* have a wide appeal because it is the most inclusive of the theatre arts, embracing as it does dancing, mime, music, scenic accessories. But it will never achieve a mass audience, it will never be great, until it finds its themes in reality, either in the present world of events, or, if it chooses to work with historical material, in the field of keen interpretive history, or in the rich traditional folk material of the world. The reaction of the audience to the ballets presented at the Stadium is proof of this. The ballets were received very unenthusiastically. The general apathy was only slightly disturbed by a weak applause for occasional technical feats. (It is a compliment to the modern dance that the sequence of a number is never broken by the intrusion of applause rendered for mere acrobatics.) The theatre may be the legitimate home of fantasy, but only that fantasy deeply rooted in the earth can make an audience part of it.

Despite the new activities of ballet, the Monte Carlo Ballet Russe, the Fokine Ballets, the American Ballet Company, despite the backing of wealthy patrons, ballet will not live unless its directors and choreographers are willing to forego their courtly dreams of the nineteenth century. The *Alma Mater* work presented by the American Ballet, a careful satire on college life, caught a vibrant reaction from the audience that none of the *Reminiscence* ballets were able to do. Both choreographed by Balanchine, the former spoke to the audience in contemporary terms, whereas the latter tried unavailingly to carry it back to an atmosphere of gilded halls and purple clad page boys--an atmosphere with which it could feel no bond whatsoever.

Moreover, the ballet organizations will have to wake up intellectually before they can develop further. The following quotation from Moliere actually appears in the American Ballet Program sold at the Stadium (25c and worth it for the laugh). It is inconceivable that Moliere's satire should be cited as a serious credo in the year 1935:

"All the ills of mankind, all the tragic misfortunes that fill the history books, all political blunders, all the failures of great commanders, have arisen merely from lack of skill in *dancing*...

"When a man has been guilty of a mistake, either in ordering his own affairs, or in directing those of the State, or in commanding an army, do we not always say: So-and-so has made a false step in this affair?...

"And can making a false step derive from anything but a lack of skill in *dancing?*"

Moliere. *Le Bourgeois Gentilhomme.* Wouldn't it have been wonderful to have prevented the tragic misfortune of fascism by teaching Hitler to delicately point his toes, or Mussolini to change his military stride to the flowing walk of Duncan? Of course, we might try to teach them to leap backwards from Ethiopia!

Fokine, Balanchine, Massine--you must forget the past that served its formal purpose. Give America new ballets of its time. Discard the loves of Zobeide and dance the love and desire and struggle for a new life and a better world in which to create and live.

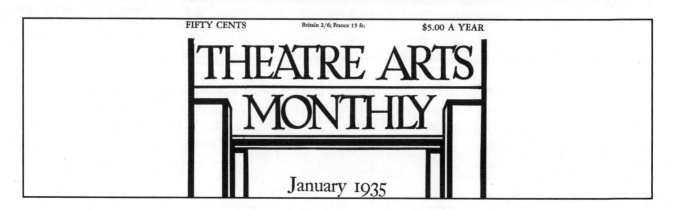

FIFTY CENTS   Britain 2/6; France 15 fr. $5.00 A YEAR

THEATRE ARTS MONTHLY

January 1935

Road to the Dance
BLANCHE EVAN

Isadora Duncan appeared in the dance world of 1900 as a "new strength and...new authority...a first motion and self-rolling wheel." She opened the gates and produced the dance-conscious world we have today. She caused to be born both the modern dance and the new ballet. The contemporary dance is spoken of often as having arisen as a reaction to the emotional "interpretive" dancing synthesized in the work of Isadora Duncan, but a careful reading of Duncan's essays not only supplies ample refutation to this theory, but proves that Duncan laid down every principle upon which the contemporary dance (both the modern and the ballet) is built, upon which the dance of the future will be logically constructed. Duncan did not analyze these tenets to any great degree, nor did she develop them in practice to the extent that succeeding dancers were able to do. Nevertheless, by the conviction inherent in her genius, she laid the foundation in her actual work and--a boon for us--in literary form as well

The first service that Isadora Duncan rendered was to discard the idea of the dance as a by-product of human activity, in the form of diversion, entertainment, physical animation, and to restore it to the plane it had held in the Greek civilization--that of an art form. "The dance is not a diversion, but a religion, an expression of life. Life is the root and art is the flower."[1] By raising the level of the dance from a physical manifestation to a creative one, she established what is today a guiding principle of the modern dance: that movement be used never for its own sake, never as a physical expression, never as a *tour de force* of time, space, or body-mechanics, but that it be used always to *express something*. "Movement and culture of his body form the aim of the gymnast; for the dancer they are only the means. Thus the body itself must be forgotten, for it is only a harmonious and well-adapted instrument whose movements express not only the movements of the body as in gymnastics but also the thoughts and feelings of a soul." The use of elevation can demonstrate this point. Certainly the physical elevation of the ballet dancers was far superior to Duncan's. They could not only leap much higher than she, but they could do wonderful "tricks" while in the air. Their only concern was one of virtuosity. To Duncan, this was significant of the ballet's decadent use of movement. To her, elevation was a direct expression of the close union between the dancer and the natural forces underlying movement; gravity and air, depth and height. Elevation was only a means to a great spiritual experience made possible through the physical activity ; the experience of flight about which Da Vinci dreamed and Nietzsche rhapsodized.

Let it not be understood that Duncan espoused the cause of sentimental "self-expression" dancing of which she is so often and so unjustly accused. In her writings we find many indications that she wished to make the new dance an art form, necessarily subjecting it to the "controlling influence of form". "But with its freedom, its accordance with natural movement, there was always design too--even in nature you find sure, even rigid design." Nothing in the composition of the dance

[1]Duncan: *The Art of the Dance*

must be "left to chance". Form immediately implied knowledge of and skill in the use of the instrument. "Since I was a child I have spent twenty years of incessant labor in the service of my art, a large part of that time being devoted to technical training." Technique, yes; but technique used *as a means only* and subservient to the *desire* for expression. The ballet's concept of body skill as an end in itself was destroyed and new values created for technique.

Isadora sought the *realization* of that expression through movement itself. The ballet had used pantomime to express both thought and emotion, using the dancing as an interlude to tie up the fragments of pantomime; or from another viewpoint, the pantomime was used to separate the various displays of technical virtuosity in the form of *pas seul, pas de quarte,* etc. Isadora, for the first time in centuries, utilized abstract movement to carry the message of the dancer, making that movement *the* dance rather than a segment of the whole choreography. Body movement and movement of the whole body became the sole medium of the dance.

Movement, by freeing itself from pantomime, at the same time freed itself from representationalism. The dancer need no longer "tell a story" in the dance. She was free to compose dance movement as a musician might compose music. She was able to express the *essence* of emotion rather than the realistic portraiture of emotion to which the ballet had been limited.

In 1905, Duncan danced in St. Petersburg and sowed the seed which later flowered in the then radically modern productions of Diaghileff. Fokine violently disapproved of her lack of virtuosity (the ballet dancers were not sensitive enough to understand that by the very nature of her revolt she had to break with everything for which the ballet then stood); nevertheless, he had vision enough to sense her message and take from it what he could constructively apply to his own tradition. "He broke away from the academic form of Petipa in that he used the whole body and broke the rigidity of movement. He used the hands, the arms, the torso, where before only the legs moved. The subject danced is no longer a pretext, but the foundation upon which the whole ballet is built. The music used is in a more intimate relation to the dance than ever before."[2]

Duncan's influence on the ballet transmitted through Fokine is best expressed by him in his "credo" sent to the tradition-bound management of the Russian Imperial Ballet. "...It is impossible to form combinations of ready-made steps; one must create an expression to fit the subject at hand...Conventional gesture can only be used when the style of the ballet demands it. Gestures of the hand alone must be replaced by gestures of the whole body...there must be an unbroken alliance between dancing and...music...Special ballet music is not required. Music of nearly any fluency can be accepted." This was too much for the Mariinsky. Fokine, less interested in convincing them than in an opportunity to apply his new theories left Russia with Diaghileff.

In 1909, four years after Duncan's Russian tour, the first performance of the Diaghileff Ballet took place in Paris. By its very act of departure from the Imperial school, it manifested its rebellion against the old forms, and its debt to Isadora. She had not only shown them a new dance; she had shown them that dancing can exist in its own right. "It was the first time that Paris was prepared to watch a whole evening of ballet divorced from opera or spoken dramatic interludes." Fokine "had made out of the ballet (*Petrouchka*) an actual danced tragedy...not a pantomime, but a drama where words were gestures and the chorus group movements. Instead of the faces of the dancers being set in rigid smiles, they actually moved, gave expression to desire and grief." Tradition had been broken from within the ranks. The complete use of every part of the body was finally recognized by the ballet master who had been brought up to think, in true ballet style, of a dancer's movements as being concentrated in the legs alone. Pantomime was not discarded, but Fokine recognized that expressive gesture had to flow through the whole body, and not limit itself to one part, like the hands. The chain was being forged; Duncan, Fokine, --and then Nijinsky, the first real merger of the old with the new.

[2]Nijinska: *Nijinsky*

It is a common fallacy to regard the modern dance as having dropped out of a clear sky after the war. it is not remembered that Nijinsky, the artist, the choreographer, the visionary, the philosopher, was not only the supreme culmination of everything the ballet had to offer to the dance, but also the complete nucleus of what later manifested itself in the work of Wigman and Graham in the modern dance, and of Kurt Jooss in the new ballet. Duncan had discarded the ballet in toto; Fokine had invested the ballet with the revolutionary spirit of Duncan; Nijinsky retained what was basic in the ballet, creating at the same time a new approach to the technique of the instrument, medium, and art form.

He separated the *science* of the ballet from its academic *style*. For instance, he understood that the principle of the turned-out leg was universal in application, whereas the style of the "five positions" was arbitrary and academic and had limited the whole form of the ballet dance for centuries. He added to the five fundamentals, foot positions in a straight line. He composed exercises for the arms, hands (even fingers), shoulders and head. He went a step further than Duncan in his completely unbiased approach to body-mechanics. He brought the pattern of movement equally well under the complete domination of the idea to be expressed. The romanticism of Duncan, symbolized perhaps by her constant reference to the curve, the wave in nature, evolved into Nijinsky's new approach to movement: "Any imaginable movement is good in dancing if it suits the idea which is its subject..." He supplanted the body curves of the ballet and of Duncan with straight lines and angles. "he showed that what might first be thought to be ugliness and primitivism can be as perfect a form of expression as the far too easily accepted beauty and charm. He took crude movements on purpose, to change our conception fundamentally. Every movement can be made art; all movements are possible if they are in harmony with the basic truth of the conception, even in their most violent and dissonant gestures."

Finally, Nijinsky constructed the bridge between the emotional renaissance of Duncan's dance and the intellectual maturity of the current dance: he used *movement* (not pantomime) not only to express the general emotions as Duncan had done, but compelled it as well to the expression of definite idea. Furthermore, he completely correlated the Duncan concept of pure movement with the ballet elements of the theatre-dance, which fifteen years later Kurt Jooss realized so inspiringly in *The Green Table*.

No one knows how the process of our contemporary dance would have been accelerated had Nijinsky been able to continue his career. We cannot gauge the loss of this prophet to the dance. In 1918 Nijinsky was forced to cease work. In 1919 Mary Wigman made her first solo appearance in Europe, and in 1926 Martha Graham in America. In Nijinsky we saw the first merger of tradition with the modern approach. In Mary Wigman we find a new integration--a synthesis of all the most vital elements of the art of dance developed from 1900 to 1918. Her main contribution to the dance lay in her desire to free the dance from those elements that prevented it from existing in its own right. She did not wish primarily to eliminate theatre elements from the dance, but she did wish to make these elements subservient to the dance and in themselves unobtrusive. Costume was utilized merely to help create the picture of the dance theme. Accompaniment, too, was controlled by the form and content of the choreography. The percussive values of the accompaniment often played a more important role than the melodic qualities of the sound. The subject matter was not limited merely to the emotions or intentionally abstract or narrative. Perhaps the best means of explaining the principle of creation and the integration for which Wigman stands is to quote Wigman herself: "Charged as I frequently am with 'freeing' the dance from music, the question often arises, what can be the source and basic structure of my own dancing? I cannot defines its principles more clearly than to say that the fundamental idea of any creation arises in me or, rather, out of me as a completely independent dance theme. This theme, however primitive or obscure at first, already contains its own development and alone dictates its singular and logical sequence. What I feel as the germinal source of any dance may be compared perhaps to the melodic or rhythmic 'subject; as it is first conceived by a composer, or to the compelling image that haunts a poet. But beyond that I can draw no parallels. In working out a dance I do not follow the models of any other art, nor have I evolved a general routine for my own. Each dance is unique and free, a separate organism whose form is self-determined. Neither is my dancing abstract, in intention at any rate, for its origin is not in the mind. My dance flows rather from certain states of being, different stages of vitality which release in me a varying play of the emotions, and in themselves dictate the distinguishing atmospheres of the dances."[3] It is interesting to see that at last the dance arrives at problems of *creation* itself, having passed through the birth-pangs of *motivation* and *means* of creation. It is taken for granted that the body is the instrument, the means movement, the end creative form.

Despite all the apparent chaos in the dance world, every step has been logical. It might all have been plotted on a graph back in 1900. Wigman. like Nijinsky, completes a cycle and at the same time holds within her work the germ of what is to be.

We must transfer ourselves from the psychic wave of creativity described by Wigman to America's most important modern dancer, Martha Graham. Wigman says of her own dancing that "its origin is not in the mind." Martha Graham has approached the new dance from the opposite point, weaving into the pattern of individual freedom a formalization and a cerebration that marks another important stage in the creative dance. It is not sufficient to recognize the instrument and the medium and the final objective; the construction of movement within the dance must stand on a solid architectural base. Wigman too believes that. But Martha Graham by stressing this truth more than any other has forced us to realize the necessity of structural form as one of the most important ingredients in the choreography of the new dance.

All this is only the beginning. Just as the present is a logical integration of all past development, so the future will continue this process of integration. There still exist many forms of dancing outside what we know as the modern dance. But they are not static. Even the traditional ballet has not escaped the swing of the times. It is chiefly in a new correlation of all the forms of the dance, I believe, that we can look for the next step of synthesis. This synthesis will take the form of a levelling down of the dance to its most general aspects. The forms that today seem to be unrelated manifestations in the art of the dance, like ballet and the modern dance, will find a relation to each other, and to the whole, from which will be built not an "art of ballet", not an "art of the modern dance", but and "art of the dance" similar to the all-inclusive "art of painting" or the "art of music".

The problems that arise in such a levelling process are concerned with the aesthetics, the science, and the physical practice of dancing. In the past we have been wont to regard the art forms of the dance in isolation, each possessing its own laws for instrument, medium, and form. This attitude has existed because actually the dance is the only art that has never possessed basic laws applicable to all forms. In the dance, even the dimensions of space and time have been used arbitrarily according to the choice of the separate forms. In the ballet, space was used as a three-dimensional volume to be transformed into an illusion of a two dimensional-linear area. In the modern dance, space is regarded as a three-dimensional volume to be filled with movement. Time has also been used arbitrarily by different forms of the dance. In the religious forms, it was often treated as a dimension to be filled indefinitely, measured only by the physical endurance of the dancer. In the ballet, often the time dimension was utilized simply as a mark and register of virtuosity (so-and-so was able to execute thirty-two turns in half as many seconds); the modern dance, on the other hand, aims at a conscious control over all the time elements in dancing and in addition aims at a union of space and time.

The same disparity has existed in the technical phases of the dance. The Oriental has learned a flexibility and skill in the use of his fingers which the modern dancer needs. The modern dancer has a freedom of torso denied to the ballet dancer who in turn possess a range of leg work that every

[3]*Modern Music*

modern dancer (perhaps she will admit this only to herself) envies. The situation is indeed a queer one, when it is realized that the same instrument serves every dancer regardless of the form in which she works. Furthermore, it is an instrument governed entirely by universal and immutable laws of physics and anatomy.

The dancer of the future will need to envy no one. Her technical training will be so broad, impersonal, inclusive, that she will be *master* of her instrument. Every part of the body will in training undergo reconditioning; every joint will learn flexibility and every muscle resiliency. A basic technique of *body-mechanics* will replace the prejudiced techniques of today; and coinciding with that we will reach a point where *movement-mechanics* will be scientifically analyzed and formulated into general laws. The future dancer's body will no longer be a slave to a "system of technique" or an individual "theory" of movement-mechanics. The scientific developments of the dance of the past will be incorporated with the principles discovered today, and those with the research of the future. the scientific contributions of the ballet, such as its laws governing body action in "turns"; the mains movement principle of the Wigman method, "swing"; the "tension and release" principle of Martha Graham--all these theories of movement-mechanics will be boiled down in the melting-pot of the *science* of dance movement. Finally, the dance will emerge as an impersonal art, built on a scientific structure, and so better able to unite its technique with its creative activity.

Let us conclude where we began, with Isadora:

"The dancer of the future will be one whose body and soul have grown so harmoniously together that the natural language of that soul will become the movement of the body. The dancer will not belong to a nation but to all humanity...She will dance the body emerging again from centuries of civilized forgetfulness...no longer at war with spirituality and intelligence, but joining with them in a glorious harmony...the highest intelligence in the freest body..."

NEW THEATRE

1936

From a Dancer's Notebook
by Blanche Evan

Preface: Filled with eagerness and enthusiasm I set out in the summer of 1934 to supplement my studies in the modern dance at the New York Wigman School. A year later, again feeling the pressure of unsatisfied needs, I turned to the studio of Martha Graham. In both I found great treasures often hidden though they were beneath mysticism, dogma, and personalization of an arbitrary nature. But in neither school did I find a solid dance training--one that would satisfy the demands of a young, discriminating, social-minded modern dancer.

While in the pursuit of study, I recorded my impressions and comments. I submit them to print because I believe: 1. That by formulating our reactions to these schools we can clarify *our* needs and find a path to their solution. 2. That we *should* evaluate what these two important systems of modern dance training can contribute to the building of a modern dance training more adaptable to our needs. 3. That to a great degree my criticisms express what up to now has remained hidden in the minds of many young modern dancers.

An Intensive Course at the New York Wigman School--Summer, 1934. Hanya Holm, Director; Louise Kloepper, Associates Teacher.

Experience 1: I am so excited--I am so exuberant. I'm sure that I have found the place where I can free myself. I shall dance, dance, dance--anything I like, any way I like. I shall lose my self-consciousness. It is only my first day at the school, but already I know it. It's the atmosphere. When you enter the class, every one is smiling and the lesson starts off with a bang! You feel close to the teacher, and to all the other students. You form a big circle, you walk with a spring-like action of the leg in big heavy stride, then in light, high steps on half-toe. In this simple way, we were immediately made aware of the necessary union between physical movement and its co-ordinate *quality*. The pianist is great. He plays all sorts of things--improvises to suit the mood exactly--jazzy themes, serious fragments, never the same thing twice. The improvisations just roll from his finger tips.

Experience 2: Today the pianist was away. At first I thought we would have to dance in silence. That would have been difficult, after enjoying the stimulating musical improvisations that usually accompany class work. (Maybe this external stimulus will become a bad habit? Perhaps a professional should not become dependent on outside excitement of this nature?) It turned out to be a percussion class. Big and little drums were taken out very carefully from the closet--beautiful gongs, and cymbals and rattles and primitive instruments of all kinds. What a collection! Really fascinating! It's scheduled for once a week regularly. I remember now how much percussion Mary Wigman used for her dance. But why should I learn to play these instruments any more than I should learn to compose music? I wish to be a dancer, not a tympani player. The relation of percussion to movement is interesting but I am inclined to think that the time I have spent in the scientific study of Dalcroze, which clarifies the relationship between movement and related elements of music, was more valuable. Anyway, it was lots of fun.

Experience 3: Lord, did we relax today! The whole trunk just submitting to gravity like a dead weight, forward, back, side, followed by many variations of relaxed swinging in the arms and legs: "swinging the joints, and relaxing the muscles." We even worked the feet in little relaxing, shaking movements. It made the body feel "good." In the succeeding hour called "Pedagogy" we analyzed this phenomenon of "swinging" in relation to "impulse, momentum, gravity, direction." I was glad that a technical analysis was made. It is not a usual occurrence in our classes. Relaxations, we were told, is used to let out energy for a new energy to enter. (Isn't it more probably that after relaxation you would be too tired to let in a new energy?)

This "pedagogy" hour was not really a lesson in pedagogy, though I understand that later on the students actually get an opportunity to practice teaching, using the others in the class as the students. It was rather an informal discussion-hour, directed by Hanya (to be given once every week). The inclusion in the curriculum of classes in percussion, in group work, in pedagogy, is a distinct advance over other modern schools that concern themselves only with dance technique. In pedagogy Hanya tries not only to answer our questions, but to give us a feeling of what dancing is all about. She seems to be primarily a creative teacher, not a creative artist. She dresses in a plain well-worn black skirt and bodice, no cosmetics on her face. Her feet are in and out of the little red leather slippers innumerable times during the hour, as she demonstrates movements, assists a student here and there. All this helps to create a plain working atmosphere. Hanya takes every opportunity to remind us that to be a dancer we must recondition ourselves mentally and spiritually as well as physically. It is always a shock to those students, who regard dancing as nothing more than kinaesthetics. After all, what is the sense of training the body to become a meaningless automaton of movement?

Experience 4: No two days are alike and I never know what to expect in class. It is certainly a fascinating method (or is it a lack of one?) for there is always fresh material and unexpected adventure. We have two classes daily, one in improvisation and one in so-called technique. So-called because even the technical classes are built on improvisation. By this means we explore all the possibilities of movement (we find out what the body *can* do, but do we find out what the body *should* do?). There are no set exercises. We never repeat an exercise from day to day. Exercise movements are invented spontaneously each day by the teacher. The lesson ends with student improvisations on the technical "theme." For instance, today our lesson was built on body falls. Louise gave us varied falls to do and then we proceeded to invent our own. We experimented with different dynamic uses of the body contacting the ground: sinking "passively" into it, and then falling "actively": not to submit but to receive an "electric shock" from the floor that sent us bouncing from place to place; running into the ground only to tear away from it, or the opposite, running into space on a crescendo and pitching from this height down to the floor in a kind of final extinction. Lord knows what I did in my improvisations, but I felt I could have performed the most marvelous acrobatic stunts with perfect ease. We had been worked up into a kinaesthetic hypnosis in which we lost all fear. I wonder now how I did it. I wonder moreover how constructive this kind of training is if, in such immediate retrospect, I cannot hang on to any one specific thing,--except that the use of movement in contact with the floor-spatial-level has dynamic possibilities of which I had never dreamt. I have seen several Graham demonstrations at the New School and each year the girls repeated the same six falls--patterns which are known by now as "Graham falls." The girls practice these same falls every day but they don't learn *how to fall* any more than we did today. At least through the Wigman method of improvisation, I am avoiding the pitfall of regarding the dance as an academic vocabulary of technical patterns.

Experience 5: Until today we spent the major part of our time "relaxing." Today we went to the opposite extreme and "tensed" until we burst, until the whole body thrilled with that vibrancy which accompanies such extreme tension. The two poles of movement, tension and relaxation. At first we thought that tension was purely a physical matter but today the words tension and intensity were used interchangeably. We learned how the physical state of tension was only a means of expressing intensity--the dynamics of movement--the shading. Most of the girls stamped like fury when they were most "intense." They *themselves felt* it (I could tell it by the terrible faces they made) and apparently it did not matter that their movements did not *convey* anything to anyone else.

I think it is right to stamp and yell your dance *in the studio* if you so desire, even if it doesn't mean anything. It is one of the unique advantages of the school that in it you feel free to get a lot out of your system. To rid your self of physical and mental inhibition is as necessary in your development as an artist as to acquire "technique." Any progressive school takes cognizance of this. But this freedom can become a danger if it is not followed up by creative discipline. For instance in relation to this business of intensity. It would have killed two birds with one stone if we had been asked to choose a specific idea for the improvisation: as, the growth of hysteria in an accident. If the Wigman method included along with "emotional outlet" improvisations, improvisations disciplined by specific themes, the students would avoid the introvertive indulgence of which many of them are justifiably accused. Only by particularizing improvisation can it be of definite assistance in the creation of a dance. Unless we practice a method which helps us achieve clarity in our dance compositions, the free approach to creative form through improvisation will be of no avail. In the end it is the adequate expression of an idea in a communicative form which counts.

Experience 6: For the most part I am still extremely happy at the Wigman School. What tremendous doors are opening to me. It is so strange. Who has opened them? *I* have done the improvising, *I* have been experiencing, but it has all occurred under a subtle pressure inherent in the method. That is what I find so wonderful about the school. I don't quite know how it happens but I find myself growing in my feeling for the ecstasy of the dance through the expansion of my own self. For instance, today we worked on the theme of "quiet." Some of the girls interpreted the theme subjectively, quiet within themselves, a theme of peacefulness; some objectively, trying to make everything around them quiet. We utilized the themes walking through space. Gradually the whole lesson became transformed into a study of the relationship between the body and space. With eyes shut, we wandered through the room. The quiet became ruffled, balance became shaky, and we had to admit that when the eyes were shut, a terrible fear of space possessed the body. It was a real test of the quiet felt by the dancer, of the mental confidence, and of the command of her body over space--and we could not meet it. We were not really masters over space--we, dancers!

The lesson took on a different turn from the way it had started. We had begun by improvising on a theme and before we knew it we had become involved in the relationship of the body to space. (The flexibility of the Wigman method is inspiring and admirable. There is constant adaptability to the particular needs of individual students.) We tried to overcome our fear of space by moving freely through it with eyes shut--no longer quietly but rapidly and in every direction. This was the severest test of all. Gradually my confidence grew. I began to move through space without restraint in big encompassing strides. For the first time in my life, space became a tangible substance, it became a reality. For the first time I realized what a dark intangible void space is--what a tremendous burden is put upon the dancer! The dancer must *shape* this space. Unless her movement is filled with confidence, unless the movement projects *beyond* herself space remains the awful void it was when we all stood there with eyes closed, terrified to move. Like glaring headlights on a dark road, wide-open eyes are no safety gauge for one's vision of space. Now I know how it is that blind people can dance--and dance with freedom. I shall never again forget what space is to the dancer--I shall never again be afraid or unaware of it. Thanks to Louise for having led me through this wonderful experience.

Experience 7: A lesson on "Vibration." A pulse which seems to govern itself. The percussion began quietly on a steady pulse in a 2/4 rhythm and worked up into many frenzied climaxes. With monotony of the tempo, the contrasting intensity of the drums, the vibration-movement, it was the nearest thing to a primitive worship-cult celebration that I had ever experienced. When the beat became overwhelmingly strong, the feet and body took on other rhythms built on the ground beat. I went wild, broke into a run,--a run that was stronger than the strongest run I had ever executed in my whole dancing career--then into spinning turns, the body doing all kinds of uncontrolled movements. Yet this happened not as if I set out to *do* a wild dance but as a result of an hypnotic rhythmic state. This is proven by the fact that at times I lost the vibration by consciously *making* a movement instead of letting a movement "happen." Vibration seems the most accessible of all passive states to experience. It is a strange phenomenon because the passivity is periodically broken by intense climaxes, yet the whole has the stable support of the constant ground beat in the steady tempo.

This hypnotic way of achieving power in movement is like a poisonous gift. What you want, happens, once you are really *in* the "state." Everything in my intellectual make-up resents it. Everything in the dance takes on an unreal mysticism that goes against the grain. I begin to feel at a loss. I no longer know where I am. I no longer know where *dance* has its roots--where power begins and where "ecstasy" ends.

The lessons we have been having I am no longer interested in recording. I am a little tired of "experiences." No new problems present themselves.

First of all we are still "relaxing." In the beginning I found this a relief from all sorts of mental and physical tensions but now that I am freed of them, I'd like to go beyond. Relaxation *cannot* build the power of muscles. My technique is slowly degenerating. We do all leg movement through "swing" which causes action to be carried on through momentum. Muscles cease to work and have the work done for them. I wish we were given technical exercises which would make a demand on *muscular* effort. In ballet you have to spend about a half hour at the bar making your legs *work*. In the Wigman method the technical discipline is non-existent. Little did I think a month ago that I would be *yearning* for those ham-string pains.

The Wigman method obviously has not achieved a balance between discipline and freedom. Today's lesson was on elevation. A number of the girls came down with a thud but no technical criticism was given: only the qualitative one, that their movement had too much *down* in it. At other times I found the stress on quality in movement very gratifying. It is the only school I know of that makes a point of quality in movement. We had many interesting lessons on contrasts between staccato and legato movement, heavy and light movement, etc. Today, however, when our problem was purely technical, the question of quality was absolutely irrelevant. Their thud was due plainly to lack of resiliency in ankle and knee. All the talk about "height and depth" could not possibly help them. These girls had the best mental intention in the world, understood intellectually the concept of "height and depth" but without knowing the fundamental simple demands of elevation, they simply could not execute an elevation. Hanya's explanation was very refreshing for those professionals in the class who had mastered the technique before coming to the Wigman School. But for the majority it was futile and dangerous. It even left them with psychological frustration about leaping. If only the school would *teach* fundamental technique, as a base, its stress on quality would really be fruitful.

When you go to ballet (I hear this is true of the Graham studio too) you become involved in technique, technique, technique. At Wigman's you become involved in a mystic kind of free expression to the annihilation of technique. The shot which Isadora fired when she threw her toe-slippers into the junk heap thirty-five years ago was signal for the battle which still rages. No peace has yet been made in dance training between technical virtuosity and significant emotionalism. That is another job for us young dancers: to build a new method of training that will do justice to *both* sides of our craft. In present systems they are antagonistic forces; we must make them supplement each other.

The lesson dealt with the theme of "Ceremonial." Not only a lesson on "Ceremonial" but on the sacrificial quality in certain "ceremonial ceremonies." Why? Because Mary Wigman has been influenced by such ideology and has used it as a source for her own creative work and for her pedagogy. I felt completely removed from this interpretation of a "ceremonial" theme. I wanted to use it as a germ motive for a dance of hypocrisy. That was heresy. I must admit I didn't quite understand what was expected. No one explained. It was taken for granted that we were acquainted with this unpalatable (to me) portion of the Wigman tradition. All the primitive mysticism which I formerly mildly objected to now strikes me with deeper implications. Real life, real dance, real modern dance is past the stage when it can or should be nourished with mystic primitivism.

Heretofore, when I entered the studio, I completely forgot the existence of the outer world. Today, the isolation of our studio work from this world brought me down with a thud--a real thud--to earth. The ties begin to slip. The bright love I developed for the freshness of the school turns into a brownish sediment. The first eagerness and enthusiasm which I directed toward entering the school now makes a half-turn in the opposite direction.

I regard this period as the "adolescence" of my training during which time personal barriers have been broken down between *me* and *myself*, but at the sacrifice of rearing a new barrier between me and reality. Nothing in this period has taught me the *positive* elements of my craft. "The body as instrument" was merely a phrase, unsubstantiated by the rigorous practise an instrument requires. Improvisation remained an indefinite activity divorced from the definite content. How to find clear movement images for a dance remains an unsolved mystery. How to become skillful, and expressive, and explicit--that is still the problem. How to make a finished dance, what the elements are that make for good compositional structure--that has not been even mentioned. Instead, there has been so much description of a vague spirit of "ecstasy": the strength of the mood, the spiritual state creating an "ecstatic" state for the production of dance movement. Motion born through emotion. Of course art derives from emotional sources but in *great* art emotion exists not as a separate element from the intellect but integrally bound up with it.

Where is the truth between discipline and freedom? What is the relation between basic technique and creative technique, between free improvisation and disciplined improvisation, and between improvisation and formal composition? What is the relation between the modern dance and specific content, between movement that says something clearly and communicatively to an audience--between that and the abstract medium of movement?

These are problems the Wigman system of dancing leaves unanswered. These are the most important problems which face the modern dancers of to-day. Where shall we find the answers?

(The second and concluding section of this article will be published in the April issue of NEW THEATRE.)

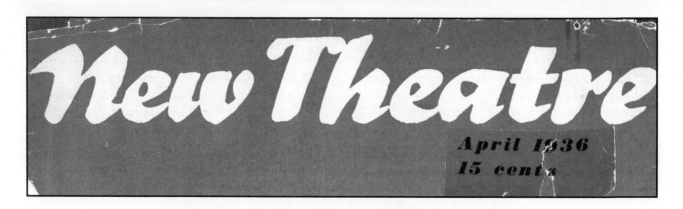

New Theatre

April 1936
15 cents

From a Dancer's Notebook
BY BLANCHE EVAN

(This is the second of two articles written by Miss Evan; the first, dealing with her experiences in the Wigman School, appeared in the March issue of New Theatre. *We urge readers to turn back to that article for the preface.)*

I must tie the loose ends of my training together; I must find a focal point around which dance technique, creative technique, and dance performance, can swing in rhythmic unity. Martha Graham, the most finished artist in the modern dance, must be able to point the way to such an integration. My course starts with her to-morrow.

An intensive Course at Martha Graham's--Summer, 1935.

The First Week: Long before class begins each day, there is a hush in the studio comparable only to the tense moment before a curtain rise in the theatre. The girls quietly seat themselves on the floor and begin to stretch. I don't dare fling a "hello" to a classmate across the room. It would seem out of keeping in this solemn atmosphere. Martha enters dressed in a beautifully designed costume of white silk wearing white fur slippers to match. It's only eleven a.m. but she has already completed her private rehearsal and practise period. She quietly reclines on the divan, wraps a thin blanket around her, one of the three studio dachshunds snuggles in beside her, and the class commences. The first somber percussive chord on the piano intensifies this restrained atmosphere. We begin the famous Graham stretches.

Seated on the floor, with legs stretched wide, we are impelled head-first into a series of complicated shapes stretching every single muscle the body possesses. The body is placed in such a position that it becomes imperative to use intense muscular power to get you from one position to another. The terminology for the torso positions consists of three words: "release, contraction, forced release." Martha's explanation was very cryptic: "these body positions were derived from a state of breath, though in actuality they have nothing to do with breathing." We are not given any fundamental preparatory work on these spinal movements. We are immediately presented with the problem of executing difficult exercise-forms based on these three positions. There is no gradual progression from the simple to the difficult. And I am very much amazed to find out, upon investigation, that the beginners, people who have never danced before, are given these same complex and strenuous exercises.

This lack of progression in technique really shocks me. Even we, who have had past training, find the work too extreme. For instance each day another girl complains (in the dressing-room) of over-stretched tendons around the knee. The students are very queer. They wouldn't dream of telling Martha this nor of even discussing objectively with her the good, and any possibility of bad, in these exercise-forms. And yet, when I go to Martha after class with doubts, she seems willing enough to enter into discussion. I think if the students treated her as a human being rather than as a goddess, many barriers that now exist between teacher and student would be removed.

The Second Week: We're off the floor now. We've arrived at the next series of exercises in which we stand in one place. Each series is worked out to set counts which are religiously adhered to. Many of the exercises are pure ballet in principle: the turn-out, the slow plie (knee-bend), battements (kicks), leg extensions, elevations, etc. Some of these are given in pure ballet form, others have been changed to combine odd co-ordinations of the torso with the legs. It is interesting that Martha Graham, the most influential modern dancer of the day should be so influenced by the ballet. Even the arm positions in the exercises are variations of the five ballet arm positions. Perhaps eventually Martha will also incorporate into the technique some of ballet "allegro"--fast movement concerning big areas of space and fast transitions between movements. The only way we move through space is in the Graham pattern of the walk, the run, and the leap.

Not the slightest deviation from these patterns is permitted. Why these are the only "correct" ways to perform these activities, we are not told. I ask girls who have been with Martha for years the why and wherefore of a Graham law, and they say, "There is no reason. This *is* the way to leap. Martha says so." Maybe Martha has reasons for this seeming dogma; she seems so convinced herself; but if so, I should like to *know* them.

Through all the work, standing, or sitting, the head must be up, parallel with the ceiling, ("There is only one point which is up--directly above the head, everything else is 'thinking up'"), down, parallel with the plane of the floor, or straight, looking ahead at the wall in front or in back of you, to the right or left side of you. Other position of the head in technique are unconditionally branded as weak and sentimental--"unclassic." In any one of these six positions and in passing from one to the other, the eyes must be wide open, with "the gaze" at eye level, never cast down, never lifted up. Nothing seems to upset Martha more than to see a student's eyes wander out of the direct range of the eye level. She says that only with such directness of the eyes and of the head can the dancer "tip the sides of the room," of the stage, of the world--(don't you "tip" the world less by the way in which you hold your head than by what you *say?*)--that only so you can make space come to you, draw your audience around you; that the days are past when the dancer extended herself *to* her audience in rapt emotion.

The idea of *using* space as the Wigman method teaches, of dominating it through *use* rather than through an abstract tyranny over it, seems more significant to me. The Wigman and Graham systems might get together to advantage on this question of space. When will the dance world break through its separate ivory towers and meet on a *common* ground of dance research!

Three Weeks Later: There is a strong conflict in Martha Graham. The sources for her approach to the dance seem to spring from two opposing poles. In one sense she is a realist. She often makes reference to the "new race" which, she says, must be direct, concise, unsentimental. On other occasions, she appears the perfect mystic. In the middle of an exercise, she will suddenly sit up very straight and without any apparent connection, her voice quivering, she will tell us that the Orientals believe correctly that the only way one can concentrate is to sit with the weight of the body absolutely evenly divided, absolutely balanced. (To myself I think, Oh, Michelangelo, how well you concentrated on the Sistine Chapel ceiling, your poor neck twisted completely out of alignment with the rest of your body.) At such times, I feel suddenly separated from this powerful and lovable woman, as if my realistic background, the life of my generation were too far removed from her to make true contact.

Perhaps it is this mystic strain in Martha which prevents her from saying clearly what she means. But understanding the reason does not help the situation. Her explanations of the exercise patterns continue to be very cryptic and very arbitrary. For instance, she repeats often that "technique must not be distorted; it must be pure and classic." There are many body positions which seem distorted to me. Martha insists on certain arm positions throughout all the technique which she says are classic in all dance and therefore must be considered classic in modern dance technique.

Surely what is "classic" in the modern dance cannot be so arbitrarily determined at this time. On what basis is she determining what is classic, what is pure, what is not distorted? This she does not tell us. And this I want to know. The modern dance is bigger than a few sets of exercises. If Martha has found a theoretical base for the sound construction of body technique, that is infinitely more important to contribute that to the modern dance than these arbitrary arrangements of technique-forms.

For instance, we are learning a set number of "falls" to set counts: the fall on four, the fall on three, on two, and on one count; the fall on a "contraction," the backward fall on a "release." We are not taught primary basic laws governing body falls, we are not learning primarily to fall with ease, we are acquiring six patterns of falls until Martha invents a seventh for us. I have learned to execute these falls. What shall I do with them now? Does Martha give them to me as part of a dictionary of modern dance vocabulary? As a modern dancer, I object to *having* such a dictionary, even though the movement words *are* vigorous, direct, concise.

Where, oh where, can I learn about *principles* of falling! Where can I acquire a knowledge of the problems involved without falling into dogmatic ritual; and by the application of which I will achieve a *skill* in falling! Isn't technique just that? Isn't it merely power over your medium? Surely it is not a set of patterns, a sequence of releases and contractions. These patterns *must* become an academic modern dance vocabulary no different in essence from the academic ballet vocabulary against which the modern dance originally revolted. Already I have seem Martha, and her students both, take these exercises and put them *in toto* into dances to express anything or nothing. This is the inevitable result when the forms of technique become an end in themselves, when no clear relationship is made between technical theory and technical practise, *and* when no bridge is drawn between technical practise and creative technique.

Martha says: "You must do a movement perfectly in the studio a thousand times if necessary in order that you may execute if once correctly on the stage." Or again, "You'll have to practise this movement every day for two and a half years, before you can execute it with perfection." This typifies the rigid discipline for which Martha Graham stands.

And for this we can thank her. She has created a dance scene wherein only slaves to professional discipline can hope to survive. She has shown us what the dance demands in actual physical labor. She demonstrates a drive toward work which slays the lazy but which acts as a potent stimulus for the earnest. She never lets you forget that as a dancer, you must strive for that perfection which performance demands; that everything in studio work has as its objective the stage and formal appearance. The theory is made a reality, when suddenly Martha springs from the divan to demonstrate a movement. It is a precious moment out of a Graham performance at the Guild Theatre.

But discipline in itself does not account for Martha's mastery over movement. The physical clarity of her slightest movement, that wonderful clear delineation, is something which we all need and which really characterizes her system of technique. Throughout all the exercises, from the simplest to the most complex, the muscles are kept at a pitch of tension way above the normal, making for the maximum tension of the body at every moment. "The body must always be in a state of listening." No part of the body is ever allowed to relax. "Relaxation plays no part in my work. I believe in relaxation through change, not through cessation."

This muscular tension is something beyond necessity. All these movements can be executed with half the strain, with much more ease, but Martha seems to believe that only by exaggerating muscular power beyond its functional use, can the body project its movement clearly into space. This muscular tension of every part of the body she believes should be present at all times, in order to insure clear delineation and strength of movement. I think I have found a tie-up here between execution and projection which takes me completely by surprise. I could not understand why I should strain my muscles as Martha insisted when I could execute the movement just as well with the body calm and at ease. Neither Martha nor her devotees ever made it clear to me. But at last I think I've found the reason. The straining of the body in technique which Martha demands has nothing to do with the technique of movement, as such, but rather with the technique of projection. It is a principle which one can apply to any technique, and to any type of movement. I think back now to Pavlowa, and I know that all the greatest dancers have known of it. "You must be fanatical when you dance, fanatical in the muscular sense." It is an intensity completely divorced from the specific intensity which the mood or the content of a movement may demand. "Dancing is physical...Your conception exists for your audience only as physical movement...Stop *reacting* to ideas...Dance exists only in action, not in reaction...Move and make your audience react to your *movement*...Stop thinking...The body comes first!" It is a fanaticism, a strength, an ecstasy, a *projection*, dealing purely and scientifically with the dancer's instrument. In this, Martha has made an invaluable contribution. But then she carries the theory into dance content, creating an approach to the dance which many of us have been fighting.

"A strong arm lifting is sufficient reason for the existence of the movement. The audience should not always look for a meaning. You cannot help but express strong ideas, if your movement is sufficiently strong muscularly." What richness can lie in an art built upon merely kinaesthetic response? In fact, Martha is a case in point. So many people, professionals and laymen both, admire her performances, they are tremendously *awed* by her; but they are not *moved* by her in those compositions which are based on the theory of kinaesthetic titillation.

Her *American Provincials*, which is a biting comment on society, evokes a warm reaction in the audience, immeasurably greater than that evoked by the "kinaesthetic" composition *Course*, even thought the movements in the latter are strong in themselves. The superior values of a movement-of-content dance like *American Provincials* over a movement-of-movement dance like *Course* cannot be denied. The dance *Celebration* is a good example of my point, because, though on the whole it is a stirring composition, whole sections of meaningless movement are inserted to the detriment of the dance for the sole purpose of singing a paean to the physical strength and acrobatic skill of the body. Why is movement form for its own sake any more justifiable than self-expression for its own sake? The greatest art has always used form not as an end in itself but as a means with which better to express significant ideas.

Why cannot we apply Martha Graham's command over physical movement to the expression of vital ideas? Why must movement be used meaninglessly as padding in a dance? The modern dance revolted from the ballet because it wanted to go beyond virtuosity, it wanted to express ideas and emotions in movement, through movement. It is sophisticated these days to pooh-pooh Duncan. It might be a good check on modern dancers to return periodically to her "Art of the Dance" and to recall the raison-d'être of the modern dance.

The course is coming to an end. It has been very instructive and very stimulating. There is much here that as a professional I can utilize. But there is much which, if I am honest, I must discard. Many young dancers like myself desire clarity of form, but not only of the physical form. We are equally concerned with the intention which we feel must lie behind movement. The dance is embarking on a new kind of realism that will carry it out of the curtained seclusion of the select concert, out to people, out into reality.

A year ago I asked of the Wigman method as today I ask of the Graham method: Where is the truce between discipline and freedom? What is the relation between basic technique and creative technique, between free improvisation and formal composition? What is the relation between the modern dance and specific content, between movement that says something clearly and communicatively to an audience--between that and the abstract medium of movement?

These are problems the Graham system of dancing leaves unanswered. These are the most important problems which face the modern dancers of today. Where shall we find the answers? We cannot forever travel back and forth among systems that can no longer satisfy our specific needs, technically and creatively. We must clarify these needs, and, in relation to them, take of these existing systems what can benefit us. We must objectively discard the rest. We must open new paths of source material to the dance. It is for us to begin to build an edifice that will more completely meet the demands of the young, experimental, social-minded dancers of today.

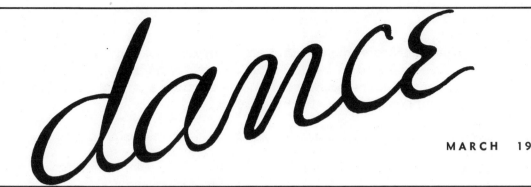

dance

25¢

MARCH 1937

a dancer and teacher who has made her own films tells
what a practical help it can be to see yourself...

...AS OTHERS SEE YOU
By BLANCHE EVAN

Imagine rushing to the library after a matinee of the Monte Carlo and asking the librarian for the use of the projection room.

"May I have the film of Adolph Bolm in *Scheherazade?* I'd like to compare it with Shabelevsky's performance of the same role."

Mere fantasy, unfortunately. But there is every reason to believe that in the not-too-distant future every dance library, every dance center *and* every dance studio in the country will boast a projector and films of dancing.

Why not? The cost of materials for a one-reel 16 mm. film, lasting fifteen minutes, is approximately $30. A year-and-a-half ago Lionel Berman, David Wolff and I produced *Film Studies of the Dance*, the first dance film of its kind, at this nominal cost.

What would we give to be able to see film revivals of Martha Graham's old dances, *Strike* and *Steerage?* How invaluable it would be to have a record of her first solo compositions, *Tanagara* and *Fragilite*, in which she utilized the liquid, flowing movement she negates today.

What if teachers were able to have, ready to hand, such reels of the work of Harriet Hoctor, Paul Draper and many others whose methods they could then study at leisure?

The need for an adequate method of perpetuation has been felt in the dance world literally for centuries. And one film serves better in this capacity than ten systems of written dance notations.

I could elaborate on these advantages of the cinema to dance. But this is not the province of this piece.

I could tell you of the fascinating problems I had to cope with in dancing for the film: the necessity of mastering the dance mood at a moment's notice, mood and moment both at the mercy of the camera click.

Or of the necessity of renourishing one's inspiration twenty-five times over in order to repeat the same movement that many times. The director wants it from another angle, or: "Your left toe moved out of the frame, Miss Evan". Or the sun perversely shifts behind a cloud just when you're counting on a brilliant sunlight.

Or I could relate the peculiar craft problems that arise: entirely new space-time relationships that no choreographer normally has to face. And I could tell with tears in my eyes the sad tale of conflict between what the dancer thinks she knows of cinematic values and what the directors don't know of body movement--and how never the twain did meet.

But I'd rather just relate, for this time, some of the net *results* of this experimental one-reel 16 mm. film.

It had always been my ideal to regard the body dancing as an impersonal instrument, just as a painter regards his brushes and canvas. But whereas the painter could step away from his composition and look at it from a distance, I could not step away from my dance in the same manner.

The most I had been able to accomplish in this direction was to use the studio mirror. But you, reader, know how futile that is, unless one can unscrew one's neck, or run the risk of becoming downright cross-eyed.

At last, in a film of my work, I had found a practical mirror. I was able to *see* my work without distortion. I could, so to speak, step away from it just like the painter.

The dancer can meet no sterner trial than that of the silent screen. The dynamic values and the content of the dance must stand entirely alone. Every pianissimo, every crescendo, every nuance of meaning, must register without any assistance from sound accompaniment.

In addition to the silence, all the warmth that is normally part of theatre atmosphere is removed. There is no color, no sound, no personal audience contact. The result is that dance and dancer both take on an impersonality which creates the perfect condition for studying one's artistic merits and failings.

I was able to test my dance from all of these viewpoints. I even studied the action of my costume for its appropriateness to the movements.

In a number of instances, I studied close-ups of the face in order to find the relationship of the facial gestures to the emotional content of the particular movement.

I speak of this because I believe the role of the face in performance is by no means an insignificant one. The audience has definite reactions to the abandoned facial contortions of Mary Wigman, to the immobile facial mask of Martha Graham, to the fixed-smile-personality-face of some ballet performers. Dancers in general have shown a phenomenal reluctance to profit here from the experience and knowledge of actors.

Be that as it may, in the film a dancer can *see* her face as others see it!

From the point of view of detailed technical analysis, the film yielded rich results.

Close-ups of isolated parts of the body in action revealed many unsuspected muscular mysteries: for instance, that though the rib cage could move side to side independently from the hips, the reverse was not true. Aside from the knowledge gained, what kinetic excitement there was to see the spine in action, to watch every vertebra perform its task in a spiral back-bend. We've all breathlessly watched slow motion shots of sports activities like pole vaulting, but to see slow motion *leaps* is a personal pleasure no dancer should deny herself.

Maybe its a *dis*-pleasure, but in that case at least you can find out what's wrong with your elevation. Maybe you *think* you've been landing from jumps with a straight back. Just stop the projector for a minute and *look* at your back caught unawares in a landing.

There is much else I learned about my work. But since space is limited, I'd like to mention how I was able to use the film to help my students in *their* problems.

Take the feet in a ballet changement. I had two series of shots taken, one of a beginner student and one of myself. And by the contrast exhibited between the two, she learned more about principles of elevation than all my talking and class demonstration had been able to accomplish.

And why? Because here was not abstract theory, here was not *talking* about elevation. Here was proof that the toes that pointed most gave infinitely more push off the ground than the toes that remained relaxed; proof that the torso which remained stretched in the air added to the height, whereas the torso which collapsed counteracted the height achieved.

And so I discovered that not only is the dancer's best mirror a film of her *own* work, but that the studio's best mirror is a film of the students.

The 16 mm. film is a magic thing in even more ways than I have mentioned. How many times have innocent mothers come to us poor teachers and said:

"But what do you *teach* children?" never realizing what torture the question inflicts upon us. We fumble around for words and finally capitulate:

"Its impossible to *tell* you about it," followed by, with the utmost reluctance, "Would you like to watch a class, Mrs. Parent?"

In our hearts we detest the nice mother, for we know how next week when she watches, the children will either be self-conscious to the point of petrification, or they will show off to the best of their exhibitionist abilities. In addition, they'll be bound to embarrass you with, "But you told *our* mother you don't *allow* visitors."

True, my little darlings, but I have to pay the rent, and I can't afford to miss prospective Annabelle. It's not a dream to envision a much pleasanter scene when in answer to Annabelle's mother's question, you will reply in full dignity, "Next Saturday afternoon, I'm showing a film of my children's work to a group of interested parents. Wont' you come?"

Of course it's difficult to take movies of children. One must be ready to waste more film working with them than with oneself or with adults. But the result is its own reward.

The part of our film devoted to children is most instructive. It encompasses not only basic technique, but through the insertion of titles, it can actually explain the approach used in teaching them.

It also contains beautiful examples of the children's own creative work. It is most exciting, too, to watch their spontaneous reactions to rhythmic activity. Not being Shirley Temples, they are divinely unaware of the fact that their every facial expression is being recorded by the camera's eye.

Nijinsky had greater foresight than his impresario Diaghileff. His wife relates that twenty years ago he recognized the immense possibility of the film for the dance, despite the fact that the cinema was then in comparative infancy. Today, with mass production of 16 mm. film and inexpensive cameras, it is little less than a crime for the dancer and the teacher to neglect the services the camera is ready to give her.

Hollywood will never bother. And with experience to back my statement, I say, "Who needs Hollywood?"

Film Studies of the Dance is certainly as interesting as travelogs of the salmon-fishing season. We don't need Hollywood but Hollywood may some day need us!

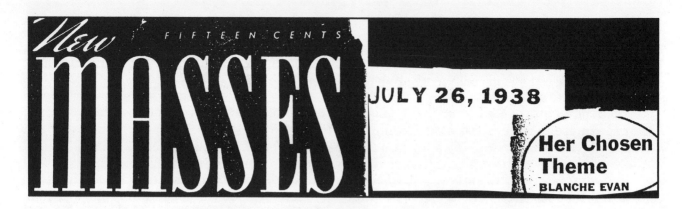

New MASSES — FIFTEEN CENTS

JULY 26, 1938

Her Chosen Theme
BLANCHE EVAN

HER CHOSEN THEME

A Modern Dancer's Credo

BLANCHE EVAN

We can't deny it any longer.. Perhaps musicians and graphic artists can bide their time until the public takes their works to its bosom, even a hundred years after their decease. But the work of a dancer, despite the noble efforts of dance notationists and the invaluable aid of the moving picture to preservation, must be accepted not only within her life, but within her not-too-old life. The modern dance, born of a rebellion against the romanticism of Isadora Duncan, against the eclecticism of Ruth St. Denis, and against the theatricalism of the Russian ballet, has not yet achieved any appreciable percentage of the audience enjoyed by any one of its predecessors.

No sincere artist prefers a small coterie of initiates to a wide mass audience. Any true artist works for humanity and desires to be understood by humanity. This is not to say that the modern dancer to be widely accepted should "give the public what it wants." It is to ask, rather, "Why has the modern dancer failed to reach even that audience which supports good theatre, good music, good painting? Why does the modern dance fail to hold the interest of that audience that loves the modern music of Shostakovich and the modern painting of Picasso?"

The glib talk that the modern dance must "return to the theatre" is, in itself, superficial. The art form of the modern dance cannot arrive at its own fulfillment by means of borrowed finery. Besides, dance pageantry has not been the only form of the dance in the past generation that has held the interest of the world. Isadora Duncan stripped performance of all theatricality. She danced in a simple tunic against a one-toned cyclorama. Yet to thousands of people, the word "Duncan" recalls a thrill in the theatre. There must be some chemical, present or lacking, in its own organic formula which to date has prevented the modern dance from becoming a really potent factor in the American concert field.

In a recent modern dance recital I attended, the first half of the program was devoted to a ballet, *The Happy Hypocrite--a Fairy Tale for Tired Men* by Max Beerbohm. The ballet had very few program notes, but the characters were unmistakable: "ladies...captains...a naive country lass, looking for a husband with the face of a saint," etc. The auditorium was not banked, but the people of the audience were interested enough to stand in their seats to enable them to get a better view; including John and his wife Mary, directly in front of me, who obstructed my own vision. They *insisted* on seeing what was going on on the stage. The second half of the program was devoted to a composition dealing with the broad personal philosophy of the choreographer: "the growth of the individual in relation to his fellows in an ideal state." This was subdivided into "choreographic" titles: "Circular Theme...Variations...," etc., and these abstract subdivisions were interspersed with more concrete though still very general concepts: "Processional, Celebration," etc. Despite the fact that the performance in itself was of the highest caliber, the interest of the audience lagged after the first five minutes. Eventually, a number of people left; John whispered to his wife, "Come, Mary, it is enough. Even when they explain it on the program, I don't understand it." Yet John and Mary had been concerned enough with the art of the dance to come to the recital in the first place--to attend, as a matter of fact, a whole series, since this performance was only one of a season subscription of dance recitals.

It is an old--though whispered--complaint of modern dance audiences--of those who are honest enough to admit it--"I don't understand." Too old and too frequent for us to accept any longer Martha Graham's repeated refutation that an audience shouldn't try to understand--it should *react*. Of course, it should react, but obviously something blocks its power to react. And isn't it time the modern dancer squarely faced the problem? Why should the same man who, as audience, had truly *participated* in the *Happy Hypocrite* suddenly find himself figuratively barred from the remainder of the performance? In his humility, he did not blame the artists but rather himself for his inability to react. From his remark, it was clear that he felt he could not react until he *understood*.

Understood what? Not every single movement of the dance, but at least the general *intention* of the composer. To this, he could find no clue. His inability to discover the connection between the program titles and the dancing on the stage seemed to prevent him from reacting. Had the dances been frankly abstract, *Dance Symphony No. 5*, let us say, John might have sat back and reacted to movement much as he would and does to abstract music. As it was, with the titles indicating a specific intellectual idea, he naturally sought the exposition of this idea in terms of dance--and this he could not find. Why? Because what was going on on the stage was not the translation of the literal idea into recognizable movement images, but rather the evolutions of an abstract design cemented with a cryptic content; the *raison d'être* remained a mystery. The sincerity of the composers, Humphrey and Weidman, is not questioned; besides, they are master craftsmen; in this instance, they had simply followed the main esthetic line of the modern dance: that of conceiving a *generalized specific idea* in *abstract unrelated* movement, thus leaving undefined in the final dance product the emotional *and* the intellectual core of the idea.

Isadora Duncan, too, danced personally and abstractly, but she made her appeal simply and directly to the emotional responses of her audience. The titles of her dances made no pretense of connoting anything specific. Her themes were purely emotional, treating of generalized joy, sorrow, the spirit of freedom, "the ultimate intensification of the feeling of life," as Curt Sachs describes certain primitive dancing. Our modern dancers, on the other hand, as all our modern artists, are no longer satisfied to deal romantically with primitive emotions. They have turned to the expression of ideas and in so doing, they have shied away from a simple emotional appeal. But unlike our modern artists, they have feared the realm of the literal, so they have also shied away from specification of material. Their chosen themes have been either broadly epic or personally introvertive, and in both cases of a very nebulous nature.

And where have the modern dancers turned for their source of their movement symbols? In the answer to this question can be found the reason for the impenetrable barricade now existent between the audience and the performer. The modern dance choreographers have not used the objective realities around them as have our painters. They have been content, in the main, to exploit an abstract vocabulary of technical movement which they have evolved within the last fifteen years, and which they originally created as a reaction to the flowing curves of Duncan and to the classic finery of the ballet.

True, there are times in history of the arts when a new assertion of the powers of the art medium, to the exclusion of all else, is necessary. Such was the state of the dance in 1920, as it had been of painting twenty-five years earlier. And it seems that since then, the concern of the modern dancers has been not in the discovery of a new technique for the expression of ideas and emotions, as Stanislavsky of the Moscow Art evolved for the theatre, but in the rediscovery of movement *per se*. In this they succeeded. They truly rediscovered body movement in its dynamic and stylistic potentialities; but however valuable this new *kinesthetic* may be, it cannot justify forever the unclear *esthetic* which they have built around it.

It was logical, perhaps, for the modern dancer to choose themes of a most general nature: of the sweeping philosophic beliefs and the personal psychological twists of the composer. In both cases, she had no tangible responsibility to the audience for clarity. Themes chosen from the real objective world, themes of a more detailed nature, would have bound her to reality and to recognizability of movement, and would have demanded a more literal connotation of movement. This, in turn, would have hampered her in the free exploitation of her newly discovered vocabulary of "pure" physical movement. It is well to understand this. The net result, however, was a definite estrangement from the audience. In the exposition of these themes, with the avoidance of reality thematically and as a source for the movement symbols, no contact with reality was made, and in the final product, there were no communicable dance images offered to the audience. The audience could not fathom the artist's specific-general-concrete-abstract interpretation of the theme, and was left to float on the wide open sea of the composer's own mysterious ego-craft.

Yes, it is right to analyze and to understand; and the fact that the modern dancers continue to pursue this creative process leads one to analyze still further. What may have been an integral part of their fight to establish a new kind of physical movement, strong and unafraid, of angularity and percussiveness, has become a philosophy of movement in its own right. The bourgeois love of the "pure" comes more and more to the fore, a definite hangover of art for art's sake. You hear modern dancers say it. They write it, and they dance it. They have a horror of so-called "programmatic" dancing: uncompromising specification of thematic material; and they therefore have a horror of making movement images functional, realistic, and really directly interpretive of the thematic material. Yet they are aware of the necessity, artistically, and, in some cases, opportunistically, of dealing with the contemporary scene. The titles of the dances therefore have undergone a change. There is an increasing number of anti-war and anti-fascist dances. But the creative process of movement has not changed. *An American Lyric*, for instance, Martha Graham's newest group composition, boasts of a fine *base* for a dance script. "This dance has as its theme the basic American right--freedom of assembly"--so reads the program note. But again the *movement symbols* employed in the dance are not symbols expressive of the theme. They are the movements from the composer's predetermined category of pure "kinesthetic," detached and abstract and purely physical. The audience seems to remain emotionally unmoved and intellectually unsatisfied. And the same applies, I believe, equally well to the majority of the compositions of the "younger" modern dancers, who, it seems, have not yet divorced themselves from the creative thinking of their parent schools.

To the masses of common people, reality is mainly a composite of detailed specifications. And every telling work of art dealing with idea (as our modern dancers wish to do), has been specific in its main content and, of course, in its use of detailed images. The implication has been general, in the sense of universal, but the particular work of art has dealt with one little kernel taken from the general mass. I could give any number of classic examples, but I prefer to speak in contemporary terms.

In the theater today, one of the best examples is to be found in the imagery employed by Marc Blitzstein in *The Cradle will Rock*. He does not write a song about the vague demoralization of the poor. He writes a song called "The Nickel Under Your Foot." And when you hear, "Maybe you wonder what it is, makes people good or bad...I'll tell you what I feel, its just the nickel under the heel," etc., the response is immediate. Specifically, you know what a nickel is, you know what a nickel can buy, and through this knowledge, you gather from the song that universally, for lack of "nickels," the poor may become demoralized.

The modern dance has failed to register its implications, either universal or specific, with its audiences, because its content has been so blatantly general and its movement symbols so divorced from reality, having been molded around the particular psyche of the composer, rather than the theme. "How can you compare the abstract medium of the dance, movement, to that of song and words?" (Do I hear my colleagues chanting?) My answer is that Blitzstein might have written a general song, "The Demoralization of the Poor," but he didn't. He wrote a particular song: "The Nickel Under Your Foot." Even our modern composers of supposed abstract music realize that the era of "pure" is past. Their musical forms turn more and more to reality for their inspiration and more and more to collaborative functions with the other arts to enable them to find a more realistic sphere in which to work.

It is significant that in Hanya Holm's *Trend*, a dance composition of an evening's length, whose content deals with cataclysmic abstract forces of destiny, the most interesting sections, judging from audience reaction, were those few detailed parts of more or less specific characterization like "The Effete" and "From Heaven Limited"--so much more comprehensible, more real, more tangible people than the major portions of the work like "The Gates Are Desolate." What Gates? Who are Desolate? Why? Why does Martha Graham's dance "Frontier" seem to get a warmer response than almost any other of her solo dances? Perhaps because when the curtain opens one sees what appears to be an impression of a pioneer woman, dressed accordingly--not a vague generality of womanhood. And furthermore, she's sitting--in dance terms of course, and justly so--on an artistic representation of a fence. And she has her hand above her eyes, as if she's looking across wide horizons. Communication in the dance rests, as in any other art, upon recognition, subconscious or otherwise, of the symbols used. This applies to the dance, as well as to music or writing. Upon this recognition depends the first spark of contact between artist and audience. And upon this spark depends the whole plane of receptivity of the audience.

This does not mean that the modern dancer must sacrifice the new range of body movement, her fruits of years of work, for communicable images. Nor does it mean that she must separate, as does the art of ballet, the content from the kinesthetic proper. (The art of ballet is built on a juxtaposition of pantomime and dance movement, depending on the virtuosity of the latter for its kinesthetic excitement, and on the pantomime for the clarity of its ideas.) But if she wishes to deal with ideas, she cannot simply turn her back on this element of recognizability. She must find and build a new technique, not of abstract movement, but of a means of communicating her ideas through movement. And especially if she wishes to appeal to the emotions by means of her idea--and the emotional is the usual channel of contact for the artist--she must then be so clear in her movement symbols that the audience will not waste one second of the time of the few short-lived minutes she is on the stage, to figure out her intention.

The words of Morris Carnovsky of the Group Theatre apply as well to the dancer as to the actor: "the greater degree of frankness and simplicity of image...the greater instrument of the theatre he becomes." This does not imply, necessarily, that the dancer must be photographically realistic in her movement images. Again Carnovsky's words are aptly applied to the problem of the modern dance composer: "The main principle of Stanislavsky was the of 'spiritualized realism'--'the truth, the truth, nothing but the truth.' Now Vahktangoff admitted the possibility of falsehood--but only when justified from within. The Vahktangoff theater...utilized fantasy and the grotesque in its development away from the earlier realism as a possible means of intensifying the emotional reality." But "The problem is then to justify from the inner feeling this strange and apparently 'unrealistic' gesture emotionally. The great thing is to grasp the inner emotional reality, the poetic emotion..."; but, may I emphasize, the poetic emotion of the themes. Besides, it seems to me, the modern dancer has enough to do today with simply following the Stanislavsky line, with just finding "the truth, the truth, nothing but the truth"; with finding those "images...linked with other images as Feuchtwanger has written of the writers' problem.[NEW MASSES, June 21.] Really, if you are in search of reality and of direct communication, the problem is the same whether you are writer, song-writer, painter, or dancer.

Such a search would undoubtedly mean a sacrifice of the "tried and true" choreographic methods, along with the change in artistic viewpoint. It might even mean a tendency toward literal pantomime--but only temporarily so. If the modern dance has any role to play historically in the art of the dance, it would seems to be the integration of a fresh, dynamic vocabulary, with a dance imagery derived from the particular subject matter of each new dance. The conservative critic is quick to write that since the modern dancer has failed to make her ideas clear in her dances, she should abandon the job, and return to the fold--just dance: move around, leap high, look beautiful. We who know the limitations of that art do not accept the advice.

There is no question that the modern dance has in its power the means to stimulate the interest and participation of wide audiences; after all, it is the form of dance that has arisen out of a real need of change and rebellion. But as long as its achievements remain of the craft alone, it will remain for the craft alone: for an audience, a small one at best, and that chiefly drawn from the girls' colleges where the modern dance is now taught. That world does not represent the masses of the people, though our modern dancers seem so involved in their immediate artistic and economic problems that they really seem to lose their sense of proportion in this respect. Nor is the situation helped by the fact that the cosmopolitan critics of the dance, left and right, are equally involved in this small petty "inside" world of the dancer and of the dance, and not enough in the worlds of the masses.

"I believe that a work which has any claims to being a work of art must get the recognition of both the connoisseurs and the masses. What satisfied the masses but does not satisfy the expert is created from material which are too shoddy, and is, therefore, also ephemeral. Only that work of art can have any claim to permanence which moves both the masses and the connoisseur." Feuchtwanger's words should mean much to the dancer, especially when she realizes that the "claim to permanence" of a dance must be established in the fleeting moments of a single performance, sometimes of three or four minutes.

We, of the craft, recognize the greatness of the new impetus to body movement the leaders of the modern dance have evolved. But the world is not interested directly in the craft of the arts. Nor does Toscanini expect the layman to sit at his concerts with a score in its collective lap. Their contribution for people will become tangible only when it becomes a channel for a communicable form, for clear ideas clothed in clear emotions. To achieve this, a departure seems necessary from rigid technical vocabularies and psychic imagery, with a new regard and a replaced emphasis on the *thematic connotation* of movement. How to transmute reality into dance *movement* (not into pantomime), becomes a new field of creative activity for the modern dancer. The "inherent dualism" between "abstract movement and pure expression" which, writes Lincoln Kirstein, "can never seem to be resolved even by judicious combination," may *yet* be resolved.

It seems to me, the answer lies in more particularized themes (which is why my own dances have changed in the past few seasons from abstraction like *Resentment and Awareness* to speci-fication like *An Office Girl Dreams* and *Slum Child*). With such a particularization there would occur an automatic departure from the monotonous costuming of the modern dancer--the consistent variety of modern-dance-negligee, ankle length, limited in variation almost to odd color combinations--and with this, the invariable hair comb of the modern dancer, her consistent neglect of the use of head-dress, and, in general, her lack of completion in costume.

The sum total perhaps would be described as a pilgrimage "back to the theater." But not for its own sake. Rather would it be a jubilant march: *exeunt* from the shrouded psyche of herself and of her craft into the light of her chosen theme.

THE AMERICAN DANCER

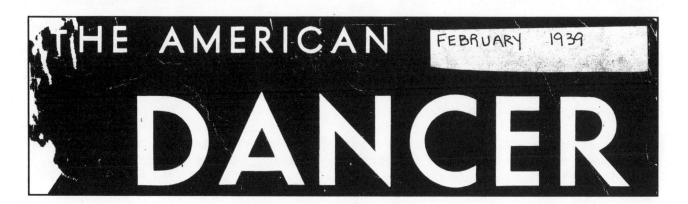

FEBRUARY 1939

Dancing Children
by BLANCHE EVAN

The Dance Diet

What shall the child be taught? Ballet or the modern dance, acrobatics or tap? This may be more or less an arbitrary matter--after she has reached nine years. But until then, it seems logical that her dance training should be regarded as carefully as her diet, and just as carefully devised to meet the physical and mental conditions peculiar to childhood. The child is a miniature volcano bursting with wonder at the world in which she has been placed--and often impatient with it. Movement, acting, yelling, talking, giggling, all merge together to form the outlet of expression for a mysterious inner life. Time and space have not yet been regulated by rhythm and direction. Concentration is limited to seconds. Creative potentialities lie hidden. The little bones are soft and the muscles uncoordinated. The concern of the progressive dancing teacher of young children thus becomes more than that of dancing *per se*, since in addition it includes the physical, emotional and intellectual problem of every child entrusted to her.

In line with the general tenets of progressive education, each child in the dance studio might be considered as a malleable unit whose physical development should be assisted without crossing nature, and whose natural potentialities should be externalized without being forced, directed without being stultified. Translate the whole into the medium of movement, and one has an indication of the scope the work takes on. I do not know of any one system of dance that has been formalized to meet these needs, though more and more teachers and mothers are treating the problem with the importance it deserves. Following the general objectives outlined above, I have experimented with children from the ages of four to nine--and this is some of what I have discovered.

See-Saws for Ants

I discovered that though children use a great deal of energy in their different forms of play, the development of many important muscles are not taken care of, with the result that the

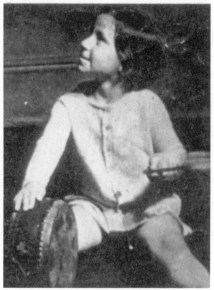

Carol

Blanche Evan

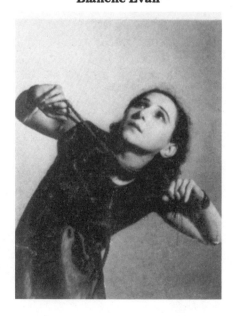

stomach remains soft, the arch of the foot weak, the shoulders rounded, the chest sunken. Therefore, I concluded that it was necessary to build a "physiologic" technique that would strengthen these weaknesses, thereby acting as well as the best possible foundation for the dance technique.

But the exercises had to be made interesting to the child in order to achieve results. Instead of saying, "Now, Carol, we will do this to strengthen your arch," I tried presenting this technique dressed up in images; a method of presentation which I later named "Technique-Images." For instance:

Arches: the up and down flexing of the ankle became a "see-saw ride for an ant."

Chest: lying on the back to lift the chest became "raising and lowering the Queensboro bridge."

Stomach: to lift the legs in circular rotation became "giving Suzie a ride on a ferris wheel--oh, you *must* keep your knees straight, or she'll fall right out!"

I found that by appealing thus to their imagination, I could enlist the children's full participation and enthusiasm in executing the most difficult exercises. And after giving a "technique-image" I very often asked them to create their own variations. They invented very good exercises: all kinds of bridges that even architects haven't yet discovered. And sometimes, when teacher dreamed for an off-minute, she'd look down to find that all the Queensboro bridges had transformed themselves into walking ponies. Then she had to figure in a flash how to divert this transgression into the path of constructive technique: suggesting, perhaps, that the ponies stretch their hind legs on their little jaunt. For I found that once the children's concentration had been allowed to drift, I received very unsatisfactory results by trying to force them back to the departed subject of concentration.

Balancing on an Accent

The second technique group concerned itself with movement principles, again built around the child's realm of activity and imagination. For example:

Speed: a bird flying (running with coordinated arm action) to protect its little ones from an impending storm.

Elevation: a frog jumping on the grass (frogs *never* land with a thud!)

Balance: a butterfly poises in its flight on the rim of a fragile flower; or, in terms of play, on an accent of the piano or drum, stop moving *instantly* to balance on one leg.

Falls: it's winter and we jump high and slide down into a snowdrift; the snow is so soft we *cannot* bump!

It is important to note here that the technical objective such as a light landing from an elevation, is made to seem *inevitable* by the conditions inherent in the image used: one *can't* bump in a soft snowdrift. If the child finds she doesn't know *how* to land softly, at least she has, in her own mind, a legitimate reason for working on the *technique* of elevation.

Raggedy Anne Skips with Pinocchio

The third technique group concerned itself with definite *movement forms* derived from the child's natural range; skips, gallops, slides, hops, etc. Aside from the technical value they possess, I found they could also be used as a base for the problems of space, intensity, and quality. For instance, the skip, which in its simplest form, is a natural movement for children, can be used as a basis for the problems of:

Body Movement and Direction:
skipping low and high, turning the skip, skipping with right leg forward with left extended back, skipping forward, backward, sideward, in concentric circles, etc.

Dynamic Variation:
skipping on the road with a bag of stones which drop out one by one, the skip becoming lighter and faster (the story goes on and on).

Quality Variation:
skipping very relaxed--as Raggedy Anne does--or very staccato as Pinocchio.

From Drum to Music

It was one thing for the child to skip but another thing for her to recognize a skip rhythm when she heard it. The instinctive sense of rhythm which all infants manifest by clapping hands to music, seems eventually to be submerged if it is not consciously developed. Ten minutes of every weekly lesson of the semester spent on rhythm exercises produced astounding results. Children only five, learned to accompany simple movements, following the intensity as well as the rhythmic pattern. I used percussion instruments--a tom-tom and Chinese cymbal sufficed--since by their use, the children seemed better able to grasp accents, intervals, loud and soft tones, than when indicated on the piano.

The Tom-Tom Stick in My Foot

How to get Faith's foot to contact the floor simultaneously with the beat of the drum; that was the problem. Coordination between hearing and moving took on new proportions. Marching in normal tempo seemed to me the simplest way to start. "Faith, you don't have to *look* at the drum, just--`listen`"--she volunteered. "That's right. To prove it, shut your eyes." This immediately isolated the sense of hearing. "Now see if at the same time that you are listening, you can beat your feet in place just as I am doing on the drum." She started off beautifully, her face puckered with the intensity of listening, but her feet, alas, marking time very irregularly with little regard for the tempo. In desperation, I hit upon an idea to make "tempo" a *real* thing for her. "Faith, let's make believe you have a tom-tom stick in each foot, which strikes the floor at exactly the same second that mine beats the drum." And from this point on, it was one rhythmic victory after another. The following list indicates specific rhythmic exercises which I developed. I could make up a fancy name for them like "audio-kinesthesis," but don't you think "hearing-moving coordination" is better?

1. Teacher plays the drum switching from runs to skips to marches, etc., in changing tempi and intensity, the child executing the related movement.

2. We change places, the child to the drum and teacher to the floor.

3. Teacher dances a movement with a clear rhythm and quality, the child improvising a related accompaniment on the percussion instruments.

4. Teacher improvises freely on the instruments, the child improvises in movement limiting herself to the general quality and intensity of the accompaniment.

5. The child walks forward to the sound of one instrument and changes the direction instantly upon change of instrument (eventually teacher drops out of the picture and the children accompany each other).

6. Each child is given, or chooses her own rhythm. They all stand still. Teacher plays and repeats one of the selected rhythms. See how quickly each get moving in response to her own rhythm and how quickly she stops as another rhythm belonging to another child is commenced.

Tippy, the Dog

All the work in direct body technique, in time and space, has to this point involved the child's creative participation. I say "involved" because in each case, I have also implied careful supervision, the teacher really *leading* the child to execute a predetermined objective. In addition, I found the lessons more satisfying when they included, as well, unrestricted creative work on the part of the child on subjects chosen from *her* most vital interests. Carol was deeply concerned with the personal mannerisms of Tommy, the cat that wandered around the back yard. Joan chose a partner to give a splendid dance characterization of grandma and herself coming home from the market; one could see the hobbling old woman, the impatient child, the bundles weighing them both down, etc. Faith had a dog that she adored; her assignment for the following lesson was to watch Tippy very carefully so that she could "make up a dance" about him.* There was one restriction which I imposed: I discouraged Faith from barking, Carol from meowing, Joan from exclaiming "Oh my bundles!" I tried to explain to them that dancing their themes meant *moving* them rather than talking them. Martha--age eight--quite destroyed my equilibrium when she announced her theme: "I am a worker coming home very tired from the factory. I stop at a street corner and listen to a man speaking about socialism. I raise my head and straighten up with the hope that some day the workers will be in a better world." But *never* evince any surprise at the themes the children want to dance about if you want to keep their confidence.

The only criticism to which the improvisation were subjected was this: if the rest of us, watching, could not get the idea of the particular improvisation, in open discussion we tried to find out wherein the improvisation had failed to be clear. Do children like to create dances? I have known no greater delight than to hear Sima--age five--bound into class with "Blanche, can we do our compositions today?"

Meet Mr. How

Do you know the importance of *how?* I didn't until I discovered that *how* one taught was half the problem of *what* one taught. In general, I found it best to:

1. Present material to children in their own terms of imaginative play--always "make believe."

2. Remember that *their* ideas are much more important than yours--even if it does hurt your mature pride.

3. Develop each lesson to meet their need for variety.

4. Balance the activity in proportion to their limited capacity for physical endurance and mental concentration.

5. Be deeply aware of children's joys, interests, mischiefs, needs--and, above all, be *sure* to love them.

* Actually the creative work never took the form of set compositions, but remained in a free state of improvisation. The need for organizing the child's activity in the dance studio seemed well taken care of where it was most essential: in the technique.

DANCE

NOVEMBER 1939 **PAUL R. MILTON** Editor **25c**

TRIBUTE TO BIRD LARSON
By BLANCHE EVAN

Bird Larson, graduate of Teachers College, Columbia University; for six years Assistant Professor of Physical Education at Barnard College, Columbia University; one year in Clinic of 59th Street Orthopedic Hospital; one summer in charge of Corrective Gymnastics at Teachers College, Columbia University; for the past 3 years and at present teacher of Dancing at the Neighborhood Playhouse, New York City.

THE SYSTEM of dancing as taught by Bird Larson is one which she herself has developed and has no connection with any other school or system. It is meeting the needs of two distinct groups of people; actresses, singers and dancers who meet the public through their art, and those who pursue more practical lines of endeavor but who desire physical and mental awakening.

The whole world is still striving for life, fuller, freer and higher, and no matter what one's philosophy of life the importance of the body and the conscious mastery of it can not be denied. The mastery of the body is not limited to the performance of physical feats but to understanding and feeling movement in relation to the emotions. Movement should be beautiful, beautiful in the sense that it is adequate, suitable in its quality, that it is the physical expression of a state of mind or emotion and that it conveys to the audience, be he one or more, what the performer feels.

Because the knowledge of one's body is so important much time is spent on what is generally called technique or better experiencing the body's capacity for movement. Only after the individual has a body alive, free, expressive, moving with unconscious ease can he be ready to use his body as an instrument for artistic expression. We can all express ourselves in one way or another, but whether the idea is worthy of expression or the technique adequate for the expression is quite another matter.

This system is neither interpretive nor natural dancing. It is more a science as a basis for artistic feeling and expression.

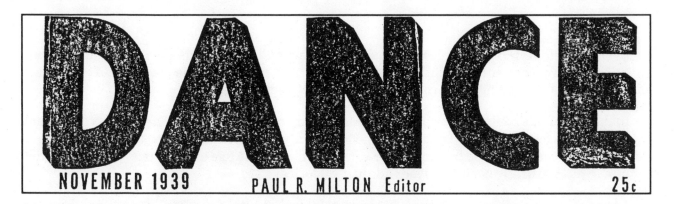

Last photograph of Bird Larson, an aloof personality whose prosperous school in New York left its imprint on what became the modern dance. Mrs. Steel in private life, she died giving birth to a daughter, now twelve years old. Larson was tall, imposing, cold, had few intimates, but had favorite students, was socially very conventional but artistically courageous.

IN the Bird Larson school circular of 1927, an extra announcement had been slipped between the pages:

"IT IS WITH PROFOUND REGRET THAT THE DEATH OF BIRD LARSON ON SEPTEMBER TWENTY-THIRD IS ANNOUNCED."

The memory of the shock has not dimmed, for we who were her students have never found anyone to replace her.

1927 was a turning point in the development of the dance. it was the year of the death (nine days before Larson's own) of Duncan with her line of flowing emotion, and the second year of the solo recitals by Martha Graham, ushering in side by side with reminiscent braceleted Denishawn pieces, her new brusque angularity in dances such as *Contritoin* and *Revolt*.

Everything in America in those days that was neither ballet nor Denishawn was known either as "interpretive" or "interpretative" or "barefoot" or :natural"--the residue of Duncan's misinterpreters. The term "modern dance" had not yet been coined.

In the face of this bedlam, in her own quiet way, Bird Larson had stood alone in the professional field, building a foundation, artistically *and* pedagogically, for a clear approach to body movement. Cut off prematurely from the fruition of her work-she died at the age of forty, one week after child birth--she has naturally been deprived her just historical due.

As one of her accredited pupils, and deeply grateful for her tutelage, curtailed as it was, I should like to set forth what I believe to be her main contribution to the development of the dance, as it exists in its own right, in its capacity as a foundation for other techniques of the modern dance established in America since her death.

Definition of Beauty

Movement should be beautiful, beautiful in the sense that it is adequate, suitable in its quality..."states her circular.

Larson measured beauty of movement neither in terms of tradition, nor of a particular style, nor of personal preference, but solely in terms of its adequacy, its ability to "convey to the audience...what the performer feels." She did not condemn the soft flowing line as sentimental or dated, any more than she considered the angular staccato movement to be the only suitable one for our day and age. The students enjoyed an affirmative attitude to the legato flowing curve of arm and spine and not, like the later moderns, a fear of it.

Also, she did not quibble about movement being worthy or not on the basis of its being or not being pure or abstract or sullied-by-pantomime-theatrical-pictorial, etc.

Larson had only one prohibitive law; nothing in her thinking, in her technique, in her criticism of movement permitted of sentimentality. Movement, beautiful movement, was "the *physical* expression of a state of mind or emotion."

"In Relation to the Emotion"

BIRD LARSON recognized the forces of technique and of expression as complementary, as correlative, and she sought to balance them *in the classroom.* "The mastery of the body is not limited to the performance of physical feats but to understanding and feeling movement in relation to the emotions." Here Larson implied the construction of a system that would treat technique as mechanical physical mastery--*plus.* She took cognizance of the necessity of establishing a living relation between technique and movement-as-a-medium-of-expression.

In our classes, though much time was allotted to technical practice, technique was not treated as an amputated limb of dance, but rather as one of its functional organs. The quality, the mood, the dynamics of movement, were always brought to the fore without belittling the importance of, and without invalidating the pure technique. Also, part of certain lessons were given over to improvisations on selected themes; and part of others to the execution of set dances composed by Miss Larson. By means of these several methods, the tendency too strong today in both modern and ballet studios, to sublimate technique for its own sake was effectively checked.

"Conscious Mastery"

Her belief in a "knowledge of one's body" and in a *conscious* mastery of it placed Larson in the vanguard of progressive dance pedagogy. It gave her students a movement-intelligence which enabled them to apply their knowledge and skill to any necessary purpose. They knew the why and wherefore of what they were doing because the technique was selected and formed and explained in terms of, and only of, the physiological, anatomical body itself.

Definition of Technique

For technique was measured solely in terms of "the body's capacity for movement."

This concept would seem to be utopian in its limitlessness, but for the fact that it had as its foundation the concept of the "mastery of the body." The combination of the two left Larson to proceed toward the crystallization of general technical bases rather than toward the creation of a routine of exercises, her main stress being on the mastery of these bases rather than, as is the custom in other modern dance systems, on the perfection of set technical forms. The scope of these principles was in a constant state of enlargement.

At the time of her death, the most important of these, as I remember them, were:

The tread, or full use action of the feet;

The use of controlled leverage of the knees;

The lift below the sternum;

The isolation of chest movement from the hip girdle and vice versa;

The diagonal plie with pelvic contraction;

The "spiral" or controlled flow of movement through every successive vertebra of the spine;

The mechanics of back and side falls;

The stride for wide horizontal coverage in space;

The co-ordinate use of the trunk while turning through space.

Because a principle was used as a basis only, it became the seed for infinite variation of movement. We never knew just what exact *movements* we would be given to execute in each succeeding class, though each lesson contained work on the basic principles. Most often Larson directed the variations, but occasionally the students were given the opportunity to create, in improvisations, their own variations on movement principles. By this method, it was almost impossible to become stuffy or stale or imitative of either ourselves or our teacher.

In fact, by thus avoiding making the technique a rigid vocabulary of movement, she proved possible the turning out of skilled dancers of artistic accomplishment without duplication in style of movements, and without a *brand* of technical forms.

Contrast

It is interesting to contrast the Larson system with the two primary dance systems begun in America at the time of her death.

Of the Graham system, John Martin wrote in *American Dancing:*"...the chief external preoccupation of the technical method is with making movement exciting in itself...She has found a magnificent physical medium for the transmission of a tremendous inner power." This would seem to indicate that the root of the Graham system lies in values of kinaesthetic stimulus, as instinctively felt and realized through Miss Graham's own personality.

The Humphrey system seems to find its roots in Miss Humphrey's own philosophy of the physics of movement: "Movement is 'the arc between two deaths.' On one hand is the death of destruction, the yielding to unbalance. All movement can be considered to be a series of falls and recoveries; that is, a deliberate unbalance in order to progress, and a restoration of equilibrium for self-protection."

The Student's Right of Way

The Larson system, however, was concerned with building a technical groundwork, "a science as a basis for artistic feeling and expression," clear, unmystic, impersonal, and constructional. She was interested in teaching only whatever was discoverable in the "body's capacity for movement" and in building that technique, which would hold within a paramount skill, infinite possibilities for movement variation and for the free development of the individual style in her student's creative work. Her approach seemed to warrant the eventual creation of as impersonal a technique for the new dance as the ballet encompassed in its own sphere--and it is historically valid to believe that until the modern dance achieves this the chance for its survival as a new *technical* form is slim.

It seems logical to deduce that eventually an all-inclusive technique would have been built, breaking down all the barriers between different forms of dance and welding their main attributes into a single whole.

Such are the riches Bird Larson gave to her students. And yet it was only an iota of what lay in the future for them and for her.

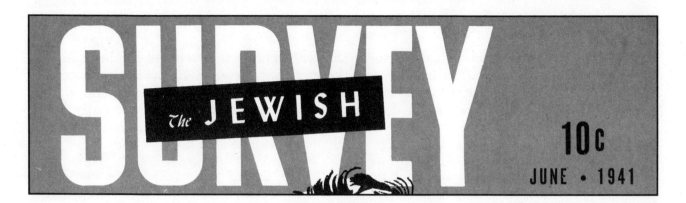

The JEWISH SURVEY

10c

JUNE • 1941

Zemach
Jewish Dancer

by BLANCHE EVAN

THERE are thousands of dancers in America, yet the number of Jewish dancers can be counted on one hand. We mean by Jewish dancers those who find their creative themes and the main source of their inspiration in the heritage of Jewish life and art and tradition. Nor does it seem likely that there would have developed in our country a Jewish Dance of the Theatre had it not been for the tremendous impact of the Russian-Jewish Habima Players who toured America in 1926 and permanently left in our midst some of their best actor-dancers, among them Benjamin Zemach.

In 1911, in the little town of Bialystok, Poland, there was a Hebrew teacher, Nahum Zemach, elder brother of Benjamin, who drew toward him a little group of young men and women bound together by their passionate love of the theatre. They experimented as an amateur group for two years in the restricted and poverty-stricken life of the ghetto. In 1913, they struggled on to Vienna hoping to gain the recognition of Zionists at their Eleventh Congress. This they were refused. Though stranded and penniless, fortified by the strength of their belief they regathered their forces, continued to act, and in 1917 went to Moscow to seek an interview with Stanislavsky. Immediately aware of their unique artistry, he gave them as their teacher Vachtangov, the noted Russian director who in later years directed their play "The Dybbuk," which made them famous. Stanislavsky also became their teacher and Mechdelov directed their "Eternal Jew."

The Habima emerged as a force in the theatre. Unified as it was by its love for the Jewish heritage, the fire and sacrifice of its youthful company, the supreme mastery of its theatre form, and despite the barrier of both language and custom, it held audiences spell-bound all over the world.

Dancing for actors was one of the radical innovations in the new Russian Theatre movement. Vachtangov especially used it as an integral part of the drama. For instance, the second act of "The Dybbuk" was actually built around the "Dance of the Beggars," a perfect fusion of movement with speech.

Benjamin Zemach, younger brother of Nahum, was interested in dancing. He grew up with the Habima. For nine years he played important roles, and absorbed into his maturing mind the basic elements of the Habima. In 1926, when the Habima dissolved its company in New York, he remained in America to concentrate his artistic energies chiefly on Jewish theatre dancing. Today, he stands indisputably as the leader in this field.

Zemach's first opportunity came in 1927 when he produced for the Artef Players, then an unknown amateur group, a Jewish Ballet. The occasion was a yearly celebration in Carnegie Hall in honor of Sholem Aleichem. to his knowledge this was the first time a ballet had been created anywhere on a Jewish theme. The movements of the dance were developed out of the characteristic life-like movements of the characters. Similarly, Aronson built the stage designs and Weiner composed the music on Yiddish folk material. Since that time, Zemach has consistently aimed toward the presentation of Jewish Ballet, with the result that his programs utilize choruses, sets, masks, and all those adjuncts of the theatre which actually make a ballet.

Zemach's dances can be generally classified into four distinct groups. One group describes Jewish religious life in the small European villages of the 19th and 20th centuries: *Study of the Talmud, The Cheder, The Menorah, Farewell to Queen Sabbath*, etc. Some of these themes are treated dramatically, some satirically, some even humorously. All were created, as Zemach says, with "love, and warmth, and because of something beautiful" which he personally feels in religious practices. Undoubtedly this personal belief accounts for the truly ecstatic performances of his Chassidic dances.

A second group of dances describes phases of life today in Palestine, in Birobidjan, in Poland. *New Fields*, in 1939, dealt with the Jews in the midst of the conflicts raging around them in central Europe.

A third group comprises dances dealing not with the Jew primarily, but with general present-day problems, such as his anti-war *Victory Ball* produced in the Hollywood Bowl in 1936.

Finally, there are dances based directly on characters, stories, and morals of the Bible: *Ruth, Prophets, Jacob's Dream*, etc.

There is one thread which ties them all together: that is Zemach's belief that one must find a line of continuity from the present to the past and vice versa. One must know the beginning of Jewish tradition. And to him this lies in the Bible. For purely personal inspiration there is the Bible's "great breadth, sweep, power, song, elevation." For historical continuity, there is its Jewish pilgrimage. For its relation to the present, there is its vast store of "companion problems," relative to those which the Jews face today in the major part of the world. To millions of Jewish people the Bible has come to mean a book of literature or symbolic history in need of scientific interpretation; to Zemach it is the main source of Jewish culture.

In the Chassidic dances and in those of the Biblical stories, the relationship between the Bible as a source and the subjects of the dances is logical and clear. When he seeks to integrate his Biblical viewpoint with that of the immediate life of the Jew, serious problems of an artistic and social nature are involved. Even granting certain similarities of persecution, discrimination and economic struggle, it would still seem most difficult successfully to present "today" in terms of Biblical symbolism. On the one hand Zemach wishes to understand the *causes* behind present-day life, and on the other to interpret this understanding through channels of thousands of years ago. Zemach feels there need be no conflict between these two elements. And if this is his artistic way, we can only hope that he will succeed.

Meanwhile, it is important that he is keeping alive the culture inherent in Jewish tradition and that he is desirous of extending its scope. Above all, for us it is important that he is a theatre artist of the people. Within this past season, along with the presentation of two programs titled "Biblical, Folk and Traditional Dances," he has also produced a play dealing with the Colorado mines and he has directed an all-Negro production on John Henry.

The Jewish people can well be thankful for this artist, Jewish in every fibre of his being, yet broad enough to encompass in his art themes of Colorado, locales of Harlem, dances of Birobidjan, songs of Palestine, the love of peace, the universal brotherhood of the common man.

MAY 1943

25 CENTS

DANCE

DANCING FOR THE YOUNG CHILD

Technique or self expression, which of these should be stressed?
Fantasy and Form are both important. Children want and need both.

The Quest for Form

From the time children begin to talk, their conversation is one eternal, "Why?" They must know the why, the when, the how, the wherefore of every thing. Their questions know no bounds. Sometimes we don't know the answers, even though we ourselves once asked these questions. Young children love to go to school, to learn to read and write, to figure out puzzles and to guess the answers. The more they learn, the more this mysterious world takes on reason and form. Mystery and chaos resolve into knowledge, understanding and security.

The Shelter of Fantasy

Before children know things, they feel them, fear and joy, pain and pleasure. Not yet having acquired knowledge of the real world, children build their own world of imagination based on these emotions. Adults have capitalized on this, often for their own advantage, and invented the Bogey Man and the Good Fairy. Fantasy for children is not an escape from reality as it often is for adults. It is the only world children know. It becomes an escape only when they find reality less entrancing than they had imagined, or when they find they cannot understand the adult world or cannot yet attain a place in it. Only then fantasy becomes transformed from the child's natural world into a shelter from the real world. It is then that they learn to use the phrase "let's make believe".

Dancing, the Perfect Activity

Dancing, by its very nature, has within it the means of gratifying both the formal and imaginative needs of the child. Dancing organizes space by its stress on direction. It organizes time by its emphasis on duration and accent. By training the child's body to co-ordinate, it meets the need of security in the form of physical movement. Imagination, so natural to the child, is a potent force for good if it is wisely channeled; for bad, if it is suppressed. Dancing is a means of directly externalizing the child's emotional life by offering an outlet through her own body for the direct expression of her wonder world, her inner world of fantasy. This is of the utmost psychological importance in that it helps to divert her from subjectiveness and ingrown pre-occupation.

Dancing, more than any other art, unifies the child's quest for form with her need of expression. Also it is direct in its transference of emotion into projection, because the instrument of the art is the child's own body. Dancing is the only art activity which welds the physical, mental and emotional growth of the child, by lending fantasy to physical activity, and by offering to the mind and spirit a physical expression. Dancing is also an excellent medium for the balancing of the formal and imaginative in children in whom one or the other tendency is disproportionately strong.

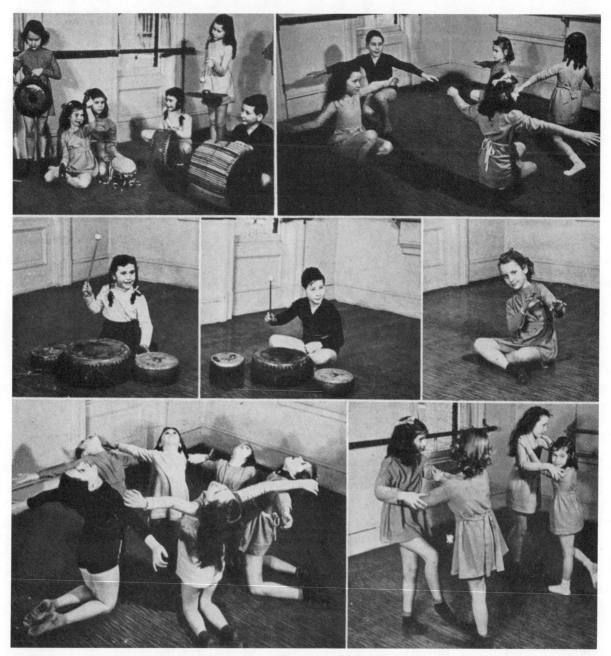

Photos were posed by: Cecile Berkenfield, John Biro, Margaret Edelstein, Beatrice Rosetti, Babette Schneer, Iris Solomon and Minda Ware.

The Necessity of Balance

Yes, dancing can do all this. A form of dancing for children that neglects the elements of either form or fantasy is doing only part of its job. Progressive parents are careful to select toys that are both enjoyable and constructive, yet often they will send their children to a dancing school where they are taught only formal technique or to the opposite type of school where they are encouraged to express themselves entirely without structural guidance. There is no more pathetic sight than to watch children who have had technical training exclusively, but who cannot express the simplest bit of pantomime or movement colored with quality. It is equally pathetic to see children who have been allowed to run riot for years expressing themselves but who are lacking in body co-ordination and technical grasp. Sometimes the child who resents technical discipline is merely lazy, and, therefore, finds it much less taxing to "just dance". On the other hand, there are children who have been badly influenced for instance, by the wrong kind of movies, who have developed exhibitionistic "show-off" complexes, and thereby spurn the less obvious accomplishment of creativity. In unspoiled children the quest for form and the love of fantasy are both strong. They are both so important that in their dance activities a balance between them should be established and neither one nor the other neglected. A six year old child can and should know what a shoulder blade is and where it must be held so that she may avoid being round shouldered. A ten year old child should not be deprived of the opportunity of dancing about the countless fantasies that continue to fill her mind into adolescent years.

Fantasy in Form

The weight of our experience as adults is too heavy for the bridge that connects us with the little lost island of the child's experience. Very often when children disobey or fail fully to execute an instruction, it is because they have not understood, owing to limitations of vocabulary and of actual experience. For instance, I myself have asked little girls to bend the wrist, and was surprised to be asked in turn, "What is a wrist?" I have asked them to keep their ankles together throughout an exercise, and when they paid no heed, I realized that their concept of "together" embraced only people and obvious objects. I then resorted to miming the action of tieing an imaginary string around their ankles, whereup the idea of "together" became much more tangible and they proceed to execute the exercise correctly.

Children want form but it is necessary to present it to them in terms of their own world of fantasy. Not to practice running in the abstract, but to run and to imagine that you are catching somebody, or to run with a fluffy pink scarf that creates a soaring design in the air. Not just to beat time, but to beat it on various instruments, each with its own timber and pitch: tinkly bells, booming drums, reverberating gongs. Not to flatten the shoulder blades against the spine, but to make the shoulder "wings" appear and disappear. Not only to stretch, but to open like a flower to the sun. Any formal technique in regard to space, time, body mechanics, dynamics, or content, will be more quickly grasped and will be more enjoyable and, therefore, more desirable to children if it is couched in terms of their own world of fantasy. This method of presentation is important, too, because it is making use of the dance for its ability to weld the child's imaginative force with her intellectual and physical powers.

The Reverse: Form in Fantasy

Even the loveliest vines of wild roses need the watchful eye of the gardener, and sometime the pruning hook. For the teacher of little children it is quite a problem to guide the free play of fantasy into the realm of form without sacrificing the flow of creativity. Of utmost importance is an attitude of respect *on the part of the teacher* toward whatever ideas the child herself may present. Criticism should be based primarily on the child's scope of her subject, rather than on an adult's conception of good form. Suzie danced about a cat. Did she move like a cat? Was it supposed to be a big cat or a kitten? Was it playful or lazy? By means of such questions the child will learn to sift her movement images in order more clearly to project her idea. If a child improvises to music without paying any heed whatsoever to tempo or dynamics, it is constructive for her to listen to the music from point of view of the musical elements involved. Group work is particularly valuable in developing a sense of form in fantasy--for instance, ask a group of children to dance with one large scarf and they will soon learn the necessity of controlling fantasy. Present them with a story in which each character is interrelated with the others; one the wind, one the storm, one the little girl. Ask a child to create movements on a theme for the rest of the class to copy, or have a child dance about something and have the class guess what the subject is. In dealing with these problems, the elements of form will naturally developed along with expression of fantasy.

Content in Fantasy

When we realize the disparity between the child's inner world of fantasy and the reality of the outer world, we can also see the importance of finding an adequate transition from one to the other. The Walt Disney Fantasies succeed admirably in this. One reason for their popularity with children is that the Disney movies create for them a comprehensible transition from their inner imaginative world to the real world of which they are slowly becoming aware. Storms, so mysterious to children, are visualized as living forms in the clouds, hurling thunder and lightning to the earth. The flowers are put to bed, much as the children themselves are, at the end of the day. From the human point of view, the Disney movies are particularly important. Mickey Mouse is quite a person; the Ugly Duckling is truly pathetic, suffering undeserved neglect; Donald Duck is very wise.

In the dance class, there are also specific ways of guiding the child out of her *shelter* of fantasy into a *positive* use of fantasy in constructive channels of creativity and of social group awareness. Children can be made aware of the *traits* of animals, rather than merely their outward movement characteristics. They can dance out stories of how things grow in the earth, of how coal is mined, of how battles are won. They can study folk music in the dancing class from point of view of the characteristics of real and different people in different parts of the world. An Italian Tarantella is specifically different in music and dance from an Irish Reel or a Russian Hopak. The folk dance can also bring out the unifying ties among people. For instance, in one of the Palestinian Schers, we find a Grand Chain executed exactly as in American country dances. Today, children love to dance out stories of bravery against Nazis, of a world rid of fascism. Fantasy for the child in the dancing class can become a means of establishing a healthful relation to life, a means of turning the subjective into the objective, a means not only of expression but of expressing something good and projecting it.

The Relation to Age Groups

Very often parents ask when a child should begin dance training. From my experience with children, I believe they have a great deal to gain from three and a half years on, *if* they are placed in a school where the problem of balancing the forces of fantasy and form is recognized, and where the formal and imaginative material is selected *in relation to age*. Until the child reaches the age of nine, only that formal work should be given which first assists nature in healthful body-building; second, which develops the sense of rhythm and of space direction; third, which teaches the child to concentrate and to follow directions; and fourth, to dance with other children. For work in fantasy subjects of nature, animals, the elements, seem most productive; also there are pantomimic actions of objects: a ball, a swing, a rope. Children love to dance simple emotional themes of gladness and sadness. The encouragement of free improvisation to music of the child's own selection is also very important.

When children reach the age of nine, the formal elements may enter the realm of dance technique as we know it in the classic ballet and the most careful modern techniques. Fantasy, too, can make the transition into more significant subject matter. Improvisations can slowly give way to the guiding eye of form, in the sense that children can be taught the elements of composition; the difference between a solo, a duet, a trio, a large group arrangement, etc. At this age, it is particularly important to keep the imaginative spark burning in order to counteract the effects of conventions and codes which increasingly surround the child and which tend to stifle the child's natural creativity. The only way to *preserve* these powers is to give the child the opportunity to exercise them.

Summary

If one wonder why the dancing teacher of children need bother with all this, I can only say that to teach children anything is one of the greatest responsibilities in the world. Any one subject taught to them embraces of necessity not only the problems of that subject but the basic problems of childhood, itself. Children are not *beneath* us but too often *beyond* us. For the teacher there is no means too little or too great to employ if they help to fathom the child's world and to create a solid, constructive bridge between it and the adult's world in which the child must find her place.

If it is important for the teacher to realize this, it is certainly important for the parent. In the field of dance training for children, parents should become aware of the dance problems just as they have become aware of the problems of progressive education in the academic training of children.

To recapitulate, there is the necessity of balancing the forces of the child's quest for form, love of fantasy, and need of expression. Form should be presented in terms of fantasy and fantasy subjected wisely to the controlling influence of form. There is the importance of constructive content and the recognition of specialized dance activity in relation to age groups. Above all though no mention of it has been made in this article, the dance teachers, themselves, must be imbued with a real interest in children, with sympathy and with love.

DANCE OBSERVER

VOLUME TWELVE, NUMBER ONE.   JANUARY, 1945

INQUEST: Historic in Setting, Modern in Form, Timeless in Content

Blanche Evan

Inquest: *a choreographic work by Doris Humphrey for three soloists, group, and narrator. Music by Norman Lloyd. Costumes by Pauline Lawrence, executed by Nellie Hatfield. Set by Doris Humphrey. Script from an original coroner's report in a British newspaper, 1865.*

It happens now and then at a play; but how often have you witnessed a *dance* presentation that held you spellbound, that left you speechless, that brought a lump to your throat, and tears to your eyes? A performance that seemed to transcend the limitations of stage and theatre and carry you into the very fibre of the human heart? And, more than that, a fine choreographic work that dealt eloquently and passionately with one of the oldest themes known to man, even if too rarely used in art: his grappling struggle with poverty?

Inquest by Doris Humphrey does all of this and ever so much more. It is a dance, but it is also a painting and a drama; it is history and art and music; it is pantomime and acting. It is to me the most perfect example of the unity of all these elements ever produced in the stormy quest of the modern dance.

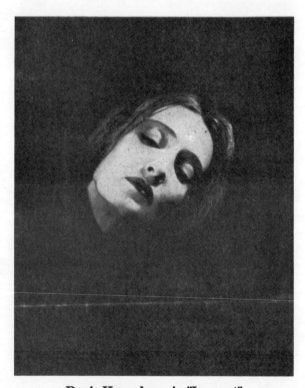

Doris Humphrey in "Inquest"

The program offers no hint of what is to come except the words: "Based on an inquest in England--1865." The audience is whispering "... it's going to be a trial--see? (in the black-out) that's where the jury will sit"; and then to everyone's surprise, the dim light goes on on a perfect stage set: a tiny room in one corner designed with the stark simplicity of a Habima or Artef stage. And, compressed in this 2 by 4 space, the three characters, Mrs. Collins, her husband, and her son, living, working and loving. This was England, 1865. Yet I have seen just such an all-purpose room on the street levels of the Warsaw Ghetto not so many years ago; as we can see them to-day in the slums of our own big cities.

Charles Weidman portrays Mr. Collins with fine projection and nuance, leading his character through weariness to the drive of necessity, and to his final plight. The part of the son as performed by Frank Westbrook (originally played by Peter Hamilton) is absolutely poignant. Doris Humphrey, as Mrs. Collins, seems to have concentrated in the projection of this intense role, a summation and a consummation of the various characterizations as mother, as wife, and as woman which she has created in other works, although by its very nature, this role would appear to have little in common with them. The greatness of the particular characterization of Mrs. Collins is interwoven with this: that through the character of mother and wife, she becomes also a symbol of the working class people of the town, of the society in which they live, and of their growing turbulence.

The group is without further specification, the *People of the Town*. The brilliant way in which Miss Humphrey has evolved their part in the whole, the fluid and logical development of their movement from the feeling of a town street, to a court room, to a dance of protest, to a dance of strength through unity, is all but miraculous. Miss Humphrey, unlike the majority of modern dancers, (though at last they are yielding), is not afraid of pantomime. In this work, even in the mass movement of the people of the town, mime and movement are benignly wedded, thereby again calling the lie to the theory that these two elements, in combination, are, if not antagonistic, at least incompatible or at best unsatisfactory.

Nor is Miss Humphrey afraid to be understood. By this I mean that there has been no hedging about using specific movement, not naturalistically, but rather *based* on near reality. The images are not psychiatric, in the manner of so much in modern art and dance. By their relation to gestures found in life, they are truly psychologic, yet visible and recognizable. The force of communication has not thereby been lessened intellectually or visually, any more than Picasso's *Absinthe Drinkers* is the less powerful because we can identify the characters as flesh and blood humans. You know what you're looking at, and in the fleeting moments allotted by the very transitory nature of dance, you are free to give all your receptive powers to the emotional purpose of the work. The costuming is consistent with this approach, having been created along dramatically realistic lines.

Norman Lloyd as composer is at one with all of this. One can't imagine any other music for *Inquest*. It is modern, yet local, it is deep, it is abstract, it is real. The part for voice, rendered so sympathetically at alternate performances by Chloe Owen and Faye Elizabeth Smith (originally sung by Irene Jordan) is without words, and yet it seems to sing of suffering. In this work, Mr. Lloyd more than earns his place among the as yet few, richly musical composers for the modern dance.

The plot is simple, although enough of a surprise for me to want to desist from divulging it. The script has a unique flavor, accounted for by the fact that it is from an original coroner's report in a British newspaper of 1865. The lines of the inquest, itself, were found quoted in John Ruskin's *Sesame and Lilies*. The narrator, Norman Rose (originally narrated by Dan Reed), feels them deeply. His *voice* is *by turn* the judge, the jury, and the voice of the people in their struggle for economic existence. In this way, the narrator and the narration are unified with the dance.

Inquest, like any deep work of art, will raise issues. Among its many friends will be those who, like myself, were utterly moved by it. There will be the more tempered enthusiasts, like the lady sitting next to me, who accompanied her applause with the remark: "... a very philosophical approach ..."; (and I thought, lady, you have a very philosophical heart of stone). It will also have its severe critics like the couple I overhead when leaving the theatre: "Miss Humphrey is an escapist, going back into the past for her material." "Not only that," said her friend, "she's absolutely raising the wrong issues now. There's a war on. She'll have us thinking of bread lines instead of victory!" These comments may arise out of a determined attitude to attend to the war first and foremost; but they do lack perspective, and they evidence a very limited understanding and imagination.

In the history of art, the past has often been used, not as an escape, but as a rich source of interpretative material. In evaluating the validity of such choice, one of the main deciding factors is the viewpoint the artist has taken. As an example: Howard Fast and Margaret Mitchell, both, write about the same period in history,--the Civil War. But Fast creates in *Freedom Road* a beautiful testament of positive constructive force which helps to illumine even our current problems; whereas Miss Mitchell exudes a *Gone With The Wind,* reactionary, anti-negro, destructive.

Inquest, albeit set in 1865, is certainly not an escape. It is historically sound and progressive in its viewpoint. It succeeds in bringing to light not only the poverty extant in England 1865, but also the strong surge of democratic forces seething in the common man of the times. Furthermore, in our own living world, poverty is far from dead. Slums are still upheld on its crumbling, rotten beams. And in its skeleton garb, poverty has been stalking through every country ravished by the Nazis. There is no question that unifying forces, developed in this war will help the people of the world to deal with poverty more efficaciously and more constructively then heretofore. Nevertheless, there is now, as in the past, plenty of room in the world of art for the use of poverty as subject matter when the work rings true.

Inquest is a classic. England, 1865, gives it its local color. It would be as alive 200 years from now as it is to-day were we able to preserve it as rendered in its present production, as we are able to preserve, let us say, a Daumier. The people who complain of its lack of timeliness might wish that Miss Humphrey had been ready to create it at the time of our own bread lines preceding the Roosevelt New Deal, when its relation to the present world would have had a more immediate impact. Yet they may still be grateful that the thing has been done, now if not then.

Doris Humphrey, in a long and extensive career, has reached in *Inquest,* her newest composition, a pinnacle of achievement, as humanitarian, as choreographer, and as performer. Miss Humphrey has, in this work, justified the deep searching struggle of those of us, practitioners, theoreticians, and audience, who have sought in the dance the true welding of mime with movement with significant social content and with deep emotional values. For this, and for the courage and inspiration an audience receives from *Inquest*--we humbly thank her.

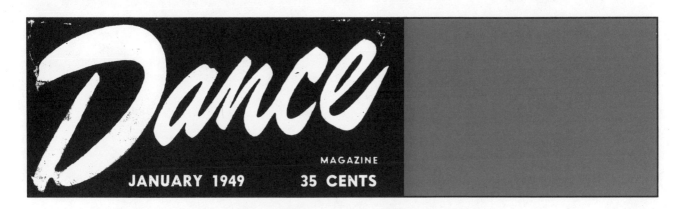

Dance
MAGAZINE

JANUARY 1949   35 CENTS

THE CHILD'S WORLD
Its Relation to Dance Pedagogy
a series of articles by BLANCHE EVAN

ARTICLE 1—DEFINING the Child's World

Thousands of children in America attend dance classes. Yet until now the problems involved in teaching them have never been taken too seriously except by isolated teachers working quietly on their own. To-day, however, the dance profession as a whole seems more aware of the fact that teaching children is specialized work with problems distinctly different from those of adult pedagogy.

In the past few seasons I have received increasing numbers of inquiries on the system of pedagogy I have developed for children from the ages of three through adolescence. They have come from exponents of both modern dance and ballet, who have reached the conclusion that neither one nor the other is the answer for the young child. These inquiries, from Chicago, Kansas, Boston, New York, and other cities, have been sent by a wide assortment of people: private teachers, college dance majors, kindergarten teachers, parents, teachers using dance for physical and mental therapy, and dancers whose interest, erroneously enough, lies solely in the lucrative aspects of teaching children. Although space limitation will necessitate a somewhat circumscribed treatment of the material, it is hoped, nevertheless, that this series of articles will pose certain questions, answer others, and serve to introduce vitally essential phases of child pedagogy in dance.

Isadora Duncan had a philosophy of teaching children, but unfortunately in literary form she left little more than a few pages on the subject. The leading American modern dance systems were more interested in adult technique and choreography than in pedagogy and their disciples automatically taught their professional modern dance techniques to children. The ballet in Russia--which remains the finest in the world--*always* recognized the problem, refusing to admit children for study at the Academy until they were approximately ten years old. Many of the ballet schools in America have been accustomed to enroll children at any age.

I can very well remember those Saturday mornings in my own childhood when, with great eagerness, I attended an enormous ballet studio in New York where there were only three of us children--feeling very lost--in a class of twenty-five adults. Nothing was ever demonstrated even though the directions of the difficult steps were in a foreign language. After a few classes we were forced into boxed toe slipper, struggling with steps with which our bodies were ill prepared to cope. THE TECHNIQUE WE CHILDREN WERE TAUGHT WAS AN ADULT TECHNIQUE, PRESENTED IN AN ADULT MANNER.

I recall another studio where I was taught a mixture of dances--everything from pseudo-Greek "interpretive" to Glazounov Bacchanale performed with a pair of cymbals. This kind of *material*

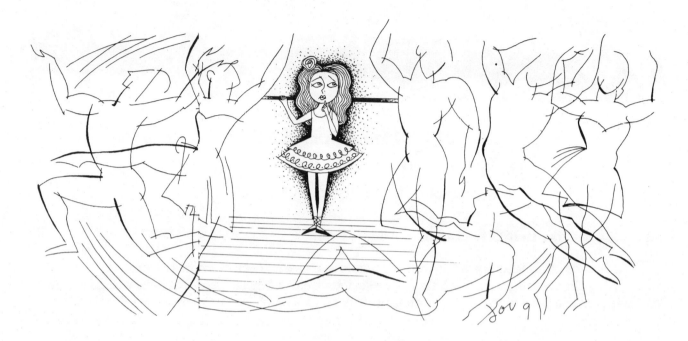

An abstract: the Child enters the classroom and finds the new and baffling world of Dance.

was more or less unintelligible to a child because emotionally it offered little point of contact with a child's world. From the imaginative point of view, it was very sterile. Eventually I ceased studying determined to find a more satisfying school. Precious years were wasted in this quest. There are many children to-day who are repeating this experience. Some continue to search, while others give up the quest and cease studying altogether.

As long as children are taught *as if they were adults*, the Dance will fail to satisfy the child's needs. It is essential to widen the range of thought concerning not only the *methods* of teaching children, but also the very *forms* of dance *appropriate* for them. *Can* the professional dance forms meet the very young child on her own level? I believe the answer is No. Yet children love to dance. What are they to do until they are old enough to study professionally? The schools that enforce age restrictions turn away hundreds of young children each year. Furthermore, there are more and more children of all ages including adolescent who to-day seek in Dance a fullness of expression that no one existent professional form seems to satisfy.

The field of serious planned pedagogy for teaching children the Dance is relatively new, just as it is in the fields of music and painting. Because there is so little precedent and so little source material to draw upon, each teacher has had to strike out and pioneer. Each teacher has had to ask herself "How shall I begin?" For the problem changes from "Dance" to "Children". The teacher is faced with exploring each, and of finding the relation between the two. She is faced with exploring her own beliefs, about children and upon what *bases* she should develop her work.

The teachers of children who have given the subject thought, found different answers: Isadora Duncan, Bird Larson, Madeleine Dixon, Blanche Talmud, Hermine Dudley, Natalie Cole, and others. But I believe all of them were guided by the thought that children are first and foremost children, whether their objectives in studying Dance are professional, cultural, or therapeutic; and that dance pedagogy for children becomes valid only when it relates to the child's structure: *physically, emotionally, mentally, socially.*

The pioneers in the field have all stressed one or another of these factors, singly or in combinations. It is my belief, however that since all of these factors *together* make up the "child's world", it is essentially their *fusion* that must be considered the foundation of the work. Each factor must be exploited, and thoroughly investigated; each of them related to Dance separately, *and* as a unit.

What is the relationship between technique and the state of the child's body? What movements can the child of five years do that the child's body of three cannot possibly execute? What is the effect if we *force* the young child into movement techniques prematurely? What similar movements can be given to good advantage to both the three and the five year old? What muscles seem to become more difficult to use as the child gets older, and therefore require special strengthening? Which seem, to be neglected in children's play? What is the effect of city life on the child's musculature?

What is the relation between the "step" and the level of mental growth? What kind of movements are most simple for a three year old to grasp? What co-ordination can a bright child of five perform that a slow child of eight cannot possibly grasp? What kinds of movements can a very rhythmic child of five perform that an unrhythmic child of eight finds difficult?

These relationships between the "step" and the emotional state are very subtle. Can we help tense children to relax through movement? What is the relation between physical tension and emotional tension? Can we utilize technique and creative dance to help the child who feels emotionally isolated--to help her *feel* part of the group? Does a child find difficulty with her work because she is emotionally involved with something extraneous to class? Should we give a lesson in "balancing" if the child feels all wild inside? If so, why? If not, why? What elements in Dance can be utilized in working with the timid child, the aggressive, the exhibitionist, the perfectionist?

It has been almost impossible to make clear demarcations: to separate these questions into true categories of physical, mental, emotional, social, because in teaching a child the Dance, you are dealing with a *growing* body and a *forming* mind, and an *inner* world of intense emotion, and with a human being struggling to find her place in the social world. The child is growing *simultaneously* in all directions; and it is this *fusion* of these factors, making up the total personality of the child, with which the teacher of dance must reckon. Because the Dance uses as its instrument the human body, there has been a tendency on the part of teachers to think of it mostly in purely physical terms. I believe that is why numerous teachers teach children a "modified" form of adult technique: modified physically, but without regard for the other factors that make up both Dance and Children.

The task of the dance teacher of children, as I see it, is to find the *real* and *practical* relationship between the Dance and the separate factors that make up the child's world; between the Dance and the child's total personality; between Dance instruction and the factors that characterize children at different age levels, and the child in particular who is your pupil.

For the dance teacher interested in this viewpoint, there is practically no source material to draw upon. She can avail herself of research in the fields of child psychology, psychiatry, progressive education in general, etc.--but none of this is equipped to tell her *how* to integrate dance pedagogy with these fields. In my own case, through observation of many kinds of children in class and outside of the dance studio, by means of experiment *with them*, and utilizing insight and intuition, I have tried to build a pedagogy that included the child's own outlook on life as well as my own; that considered her inner emotional life, her groping mind, her growing body, and her relations to adults and to other children--in other words, the child's whole self.

In a forthcoming article, Blanche Evan will discuss "The Child's NEEDS in relation to the Dance."

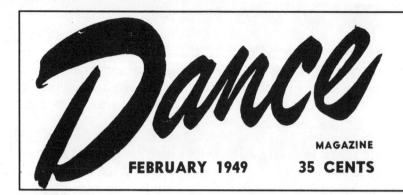

MAGAZINE

FEBRUARY 1949   35 CENTS

THE CHILD'S WORLD
Its Relation to Dance Pedagogy
a series of articles by BLANCHE EVAN

ARTICLE II - The Child's Need

IN ARTICLE I of the January issue, "Defining the Child's World", I discussed the following points:

1: The Dance should be taught a child *not* as if she were an adult, but rather in relation to a child's world;
2: The child's world includes physical, emotional, mental and social factors in relation to specific age;
3: The teacher of Dance has the task of relating her instruction to each of these factors;
4: All four factors are in a process of growth simultaneously;
5: The Blanche Evan System of Dance Pedagogy is built in relation to the total personality: to the fusion of these factors at specific age levels.

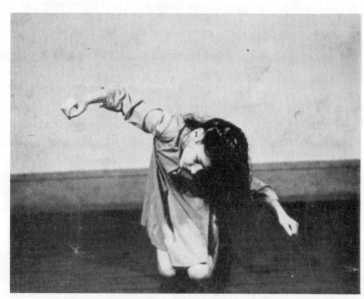

". . . a child is 'angular' and 'bony'", but beautiful when she achieves unobstructed expressiveness. Marie's own dance composition to Joyce Kilmer's "Trees".

THE CHILD's specific emotional physical, mental and social characteristics at successive age levels create certain needs. An activity can be intelligible and productive to a child only if it is regulated in relation to these needs. Obviously, these needs exist within the child. They live in the child twenty-four hours of every day. She has had certain of them since she was born. They have been affected by her environment and they are modified as she grows older. She comes to her teacher and to her activities with them, and with the need of their being fulfilled. A good teacher can direct these needs and channelize them, but she does not plant them there originally. The needs of the child should determine what phase of Dance she should experience in the studio, just as the child's needs should determine her diet.

I wish to make very clear that in designating the child's needs as of first importance, I do not mean to imply that the child should be "pampered". Not at all. I do mean that *any* subject taught to children's living, embraces, of necessity, not only the problems of that subject but the basic problems of childhood itself.

This sets quite a different stage for teaching children the Dance, from that of the professional concept most in use. A professional dancer knows that the Dance *profession* makes *its* demands upon the student: daily technical practice, rigid self-discipline, the execution of movement far beyond normal scope, very often to the extent of over-straining the body. When the child dances, however, the position is reversed: it is the child's needs that make their demands upon the Dance -- and rightly so.

To understand the child's needs is our first task. These needs are multiple. The basic needs are common to all children the world over although they are vastly conditioned by their particular cultures and environment. There is a single, basic need which the Dance, more than any other activity, is equipped to fulfill. Although the child's needs exist outside of *professional* Dance, many of them are closely related to the nonprofessional *activity* of Dance, for the reason that many of the child's needs co-exist with the role that personal body movement plays in her development.

The need I am referring to in particular, is the need of the human being to experience the physical equivalent of the psyche in the body through action. In infancy, the child enjoyed this unification. In a tantrum, she not only screamed, she also *kicked her legs* in the air. When she was happy, she gurgled and bounced for joy. As she got older, she not only bounced, but she jumped, hopped, or skipped about to express her joy -- *she did not stand still*. Or when she was sad, she buried her head in her arms, or "curled up" in the adult's lap. Although she was using movement as it is used in Dance, she used her body thus not "to dance", not because she was a dancer, neither to be "graceful" nor to "gain poise", but simply because it was normal and natural to use her body in her own personal way to express her inner self.

For the very young child, body movement is the natural vehicle and outlet for the psyche, for both the positive and negative, for both joy and frustration. With adulthood, there is a valid diminution of spontaneous physical expression. But in addition to that, in our culture and particularly in Anglo-Saxon society, convention imposes a ruthless prohibition of physical spon- taneity, long before it is necessary to "grow up". The body and the emotions are divorced from each other, and their unification destroyed. This severance prevents the child from a feeling of real integration, and creates a need which is not fulfilled in the usual activities. (Think of our children *sitting straight* in a schoolroom for five consecutive hours a day using *only* the mind!) There are many middle aged adults to-day who enter dance classes for the sole purpose of trying to satisfy this same need, frustrated since childhood.

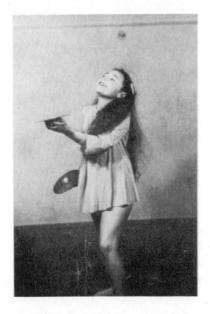 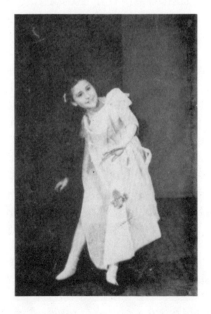

". . . they sometimes need to do a wild dance, as well as a pretty one". Minda, in two successive lessons.

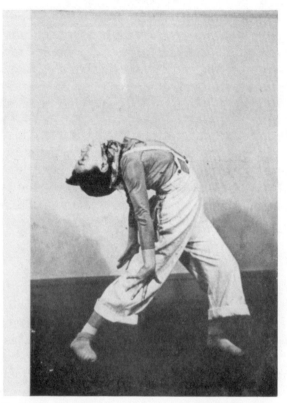

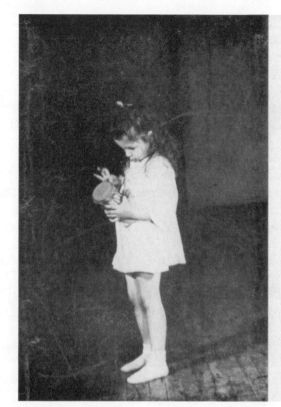

"... her whole body as a unit." Rena, aged 12.   Elizabeth, aged 6. "What is a drum?"

If we examine adult language, we find many examples of our *symbolic* acceptance of the role of the body as a natural dynamic outlet of thought and emotion: "to face the challenge"; "to fly into a rage"; "to settle down"; "to stand up for your rights", etc. But in *practical* living, the body has been so severed from its role of expression, that even the use of hand gesture in conversation is considered vulgar. Approved bodily expression is limited to games, sports, mechanical accessories, where there is always a specific and, to all appearances, an impersonal objective: to shoot the ball *into* the basket, to jump *over* the obstacle, etc., to win against your opponent in a "fair" way, etc. These athletic experiences afford an outlet for certain emotional needs, but they are

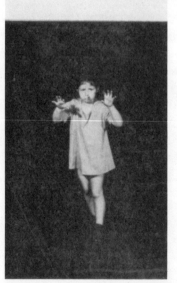

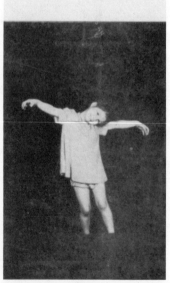

"... children experience an emotional world quite foreign to most adults". Sara in two contrasting moods.

not equipped to satisfy many others. It might very well be that the American craze for athletics is due to the fact that this *is* the only approved form of physical expression. Even free forms of social dancing, like jitter-bugging, is looked down upon by the majority of cultured people.

An adult may feel happy *inside;* her eyes may light up; but a young child's whole body as a unit is happy, or sad, or destructive, or shy, -- *in action.* To experience this psycho-physical unity is a basic need which all progressive teachers realize. In music, the progressive teacher of children correlates body movement with every phase of musical instruction, while in painting, the child is given finger paints, bringing the body into direct action -- much more direct than in the use of brushes.

It is the need of psycho-physical union that Dance can so directly fulfill. Dance has the unique characteristic of not having to resort even to an outside means , such as in painting and instrumental music. Its *instrument* of expression *is* the human body movement. The child's whole gamut of emotions has a direct channel for expression from the inner world. through her own body, to the outer world. This directness *from source to form* in body action has an immediacy of expression which is most gratifying, and has many important advantages.

Body movement in Dance can be "abstract" enough -- (abstract in the best sense: the *essence* of reality) -- to permit of a wide range of intensity and quality and of a wide choice of thematic material. Children *need* to do a wild dance as well as a pretty or a sad one. Also, the child is not afraid to dance out feelings which she would be *ashamed* to voice in words. *I could not find in language the equivalent* for the *violence* I have seen children express in dance. And I would have to be a poet to describe the sadness and the delicacy. In true creative dance, the form springs from the source; in quick evanescence, it comes and goes and there is not even a momentary reminder of that which has been expressed, be that hatred or sensitivity or yearning. The children would not, even if they could, describe their expression in words, because they repress this very material from consciousness.

A child's greatest experience in expression from infancy is through her body. A child's body movement is the most mature expressive medium she possesses. The photos that illustrate this article, taken in action in an ordinary class at my School, show a depth of emotional expression which we, as adults, don't ordinarily associate with children so young. Their ability to express themselves with such depth is years ahead of their ability in expression in *any* other form.

When the intensity of emotion is heightened, the human being brings more and more of the body into expression. Here too the Dance has an advantage for the child, because it is the only art where the whole body can be used as a unit in action -- a factor which distinguishes it even from the direct use of the body in drama and song. It is interesting that different age groups in classes seem to have preferences for certain kinds of movement, but they all love one thing in common: "to jump in their own way". To permit them to do this has never yet failed as a means of restoring their interest *or* their energy, (usually one and the same thing!). The reason is, I think, that in "jumping" they naturally use the whole body as a unit -- all forces are brought to bear to execute the jump.

This concept, "body as a unit" needs a searching analysis. The body that the child has used from infancy as a natural expressive outlet for joy and grief, etc., is the same body that has performed functional movements: grasping objects, walking and running to a destination, sitting down, etc. The child's structural, functional movement cannot be separated from the forms of expressive movements her body assumes. The body naturally assumes them because they are right for that *particular* child: for her physical make-up, her age, her total personality. A heavy child *must* dance differently from a fragile one. An average child of three and a half years, dancing to gay music, will not skip because she *can't*. Her body balance and rhythmic coordinations are not up to it. Not only is her body limited to different kinds of movement as different ages, just as she crawls and walks, and walks differently at different ages, but *different parts of her body* are at different stages of development simultaneously: children of five find it very difficult to *play* a skip rhythm *quickly* on a tambourine. They find it difficult to *do* a skip *slowly* in body movement, because of the unequal development of muscular co-ordinations involved in hand and foot.

Structure and function and all the sources of expressive movement are almost inextricably ONE in the child. That is why it is impossible for an adult to reproduce the true movement of a child, in dancing, no matter how much she has observed them. That is why an adult's choreography for children always looks impossibly stilted. In order for the child to really find a physical equivalent of her psychic self, to really find the satisfaction of that unity, she must be allowed to use *her* body as the unit it is. She must dance through *the* body, and not through a standard idea of the body, as fixed and imposed by one art form of dance or another. In a true improvisation, the child performs sequences of movements that an adult could not possibly invent for the child or for herself, because they occur spontaneously as a result of the dynamic relations that exist among the factors of her total personality.

In the Dance for children, I believe the forms of body movement should be allowed to *derive* from the functional structure. If we have more acceptance of children's bodies as nature has made them, our standards are automatically changed. For instance, what really *is* an *awkward* child in dance? Children jump with bent knees, their arms are angular and "bony", their bodies assume every kind of "distorted" position when they balance on one leg. The forms the bodies of children take, in expressive dance, and in certain phases of technique, seem foreign to the adult, primarily because no account is taken of the child's functional and structural body; also because children experience an emotional world foreign to, or forgotten, or suppressed, by most adults. An attitude of respect for the child's body in Dance opens a new experience for the adult in terms of expressive communication.

Whether the adult understands the motion or the emotion, or neither, or both, the teacher must give the child the opportunity and must encourage the child to dance *in her own way* whether this way be "awkward" or "graceful" or "skillful" from the adult's point of view. Otherwise, the Dance fails to meet the Child's basic need.

This does not mean that a dance teacher cannot help a child to attain better physical co-ordination, a problem which we will discuss in future articles. I do believe, however, that you cannot help her along these lines unless you first help her, through devious ways and means and devices, to achieve a *true* and *unobstructed expression of herself* in movement; until you have released that rhythm and expressiveness which is right for her. Poise and grace, co-ordinations and skill, are much more often a result of psychological cathartic through personal body movement than a state of movement and body made possible by the acquirement of dance "techniques".

"Self-expression" in Dance has come in for much ridicule -- and with much justification! The need for true expression of the self has nothing to do with wandering around barefoot to romantic music. To be really "natural" in Dance expression *is* to feel the *beat* of rhythm, to express the fullness and sadness of living, to be thrilled with the power of one's body, to use the body as a unified whole, and to derive enormous satisfaction from the continued unification of "body and soul".

Aritcle III will discuss: Dance as an Art Form in Relation to the Child's World.

Dance

MAGAZINE

MARCH 1949   **35 CENTS**

THE CHILD'S WORLD

Its Relation To Dance Pedagogy

a series of articles by
BLANCHE EVAN

ARTICLE III

The Link Between

In a more primitive society, the child does not go to a "school" for dancing. He learns by imitating his elders. He grows up in a fixed cultural pattern. This vivid photograph by author-photographer Earl Leaf, taken in the interior of Cuba, illustrates this assimilative process of the native child.

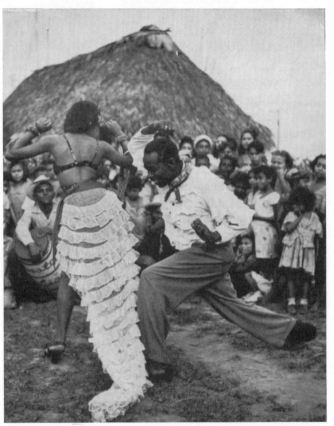

reprinte by permission of A. S. Barnes from "Isles of Rhythm" by Earl Leaf. Photo by EARL LEAF, courtesy of Rapho-Guillemette

The subject matter of article II in the February issue was: To experience the physical equivalent of the psyche in body action is a universal basic need which the Dance is abundantly qualified to fulfill.

We must determine the relationship between this need and organized dance instruction. We must also clarify the child's position in relation to the formal Art of Dance.

We assume that the largest phase of organized dance instruction deals with "technique". We forget that this phenomenon is absolutely peculiar to *our* culture. Only the growth of ballet dance in theatre, and modern dance *after* Duncan, caused technique to become a *thing in itself*, whereby technical virtuosity, as an end, assumed enormous proportions without parallel in other art forms--except, perhaps, in operatic singing.

In almost all contemporary cultures but Western, dance technique has little independent existence, because Dance, even in its highest forms, is integrated with the life of the people. In many parts of the world *to-day*, as in ancient and primitive times, the regional dances of a country, the festival, religious and theatre forms, are all closely allied. Often, they are done not in a theatre at all, but in the natural environment of living. The children grow up seeing these dance *and* doing them, never thinking in terms of "technique". The child who becomes "professional" does more *dances* and more *often*, and goes to a teacher's studio to perfect them. We have copious material to bear this out in stills, moving pictures, and literature, of the children in Bali, in Haiti, in Africa and Mexico, etc.

In our country, concert dance, in its purpose, its forms, and therefore in its techniques, has suffered almost a complete separation from indigenous dance. In addition, our mores repress physical spontaneity. Furthermore, most children have their first outside contact, years before

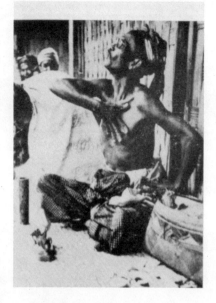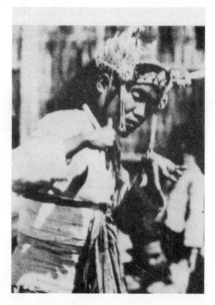

A Balinese merchant making a sale strikes a gesture – His counterpart in a formal Balinese dance drama: an illustration of the thin line between the social and the formal dance in a primitive society.

they are able to absorb the experience healthfully, with theatre dance whose technique was long ago severed from expressional drives. An assemblé with batterie for instance, no longer expresses joy or tantrum, though it is certainly a jump. Long ago it has been divorced from the emotions which originally *call forth* jumping. No one knows this better than the theatre choreographer, who uses such movements arbitrarily, and—too often—without dramatic or emotional intention. The professional dancer who performs this difficult technical feat, has succeeded, through a *painful process,* and *against* all the characteristics of nature, in *separating* dance technique from personal moods, from social expression, from thematic demands, and certainly from all those sources of movement natural to the child.

For children actually do not feel any dichotomy between emotional "expression" and "technique" unless such separation is forced upon them. If you give a child a problem of beating out on a drum a crescendo-accelerando, her whole body intensifies with the excitement inherent in that specific dynamic pattern.

Or perhaps you give children and exercise solely for technical objectives: let us say, to strengthen spinal muscles by a slow opening movement of the torso. This may be the *teacher's* intention--but the children permeate the movement with its related quality, because children will take any movement that even remotely lends itself, and transmute it through inner emotional response into a form fused with content.

Professional techniques, however, modern as well as ballet, have deviated so far from the basic springs of movement, that they have become inadequate in stimulating even the average (not the gifted) professional with the richness of dynamic variation which is the life of Dance. This alone is sufficient to disqualify our present theatre techniques for children. The techniques have been consciously developed for a stylized theatre, to be performed by a standard body whose very ideal of attainment has been determined by the *most* proficient technicians in theatre dance history. This leaves no room whatsoever for the normal, average young child, nor even her natural physical structure *which changes year by year*, nor for her possible physical deficiencies. It certainly leaves no room for allowing the child to use *her* body in dance as the unit it is.

Professional techniques were never meant to satisfy the active needs of the ordinary mortal: (non-professional): the child, the college girl, the business man and woman, the millions of people who need to dance, and who would dance if they weren't intimidated by our *kind* of theatrical presentation and by the dearth of lay dance activity. The link between these two has been destroyed, with disastrous results. For one needs the other for the richest development of each.

The active needs of the child and the layman cannot find satisfaction in our formal dance technique, because their PRIMAL ties are with GENERIC dance. Ballet from its first movement treats the body for ITS final objective--a perfect detached instrument for the execution of finished stylized choreography for the stage. It wastes no time in achieving its objective. It skips over the phases of Dance that are inborn and innate, that are as old as man, that will live on long after our present theatre dance forms have passed -- and that are well nigh stifled in our society. Ballet makes of the study of Dance, *as so many of our modern schools also do*, a purely technical feat. It ignores, and defeats, the very ONENESS the child is *fortunate* to possess.

I believe in the study of ballet -- pure Cecchetti ballet. I do not believe *at all* in "modified" or -- "natural ballet", whatever that is! However, I have proven in the cases of my own child students, that after a few years of work in freeing their creativity in movement, and in *technical work of the nature of children*, when they enter pure Cecchetti ballet classes they apply themselves excellently, *because* they have been directed to an understanding of the role of Ballet in the scheme of Dance. Furthermore, they do not carry over into their thematic improvisations any stilted forms of initiative technique. On the other hand, the children (and adults) who have come to me with a professional "foundation"--ballet or modern--have, without exception, found this foundation to be a stone wall barrier to creative work, to self-confidence in generating movement, and to dynamic, meaningful movement.

What role, then, *can* organized dance technique fill in the child's life? Is it right to teach young children any "technique" at all? I believe it is but that we cannot pluck this technique from the tree of our theatre Dance, because its roots feed upon a different soil.

The total personality makes a unit of the child's forms in true creative dance. The *preservation* of this unit should be the core, as well, of the technical work we build for her. When the elements of this unit *must* be separated, this must be done with the utmost care, else the separation destroys the psychophysical unity so essential to the child's happiness and benefit. Our problem, then, is to create a pedagogy: a technique and teaching methods.

1. that is in rapport with the total personality of children
2. that is determined by their natural structure at different age levels: posture, for instance
3. that permits variability for the unique structure of the individual child
4. that is determined also by children's natural forms of functional activities at different age levels: such as walking, sitting, joint articulation, etc.
5. that is *constructive* from all points of view
6. that exploits the child's potentials to the full
7. that satisfies needs of the contemporary child other activities cannot--or do not--cope with
8. that is helpful to, rather than destructive, of expressive growth
9. that forms a bridge between the

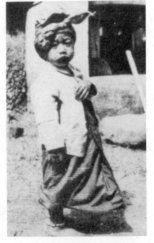 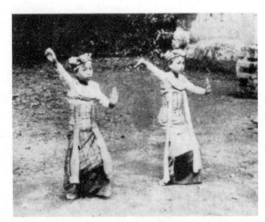

A little Balinese boy costumed by his parents for a religious ceremony. He grows into the more formal attire for the religious dances illustraed on the right by the seven year old temple dancers. Their school is the temple and their society.

non-professional activity of Dance and the theatre dance to which the child is exposed in our culture

10. that will be a foundation for more extensive study in body movement and for professional specialization if she should choose.

The ART FORM and its training come at the END of the sequence. The relation between non-professional and professional dance activity in the studio *where both take place*, requires its own theoretical considerations. The tragedy for children occurs when the child is thrust into professional training with disregard for her functional and structural self, and without having been given the opportunity, *denied her in our particular society*, of original and lay dance activity. For even the child who wishes to *be* a professional is still a human being and for the *best professional development* needs to fulfill her natural self.

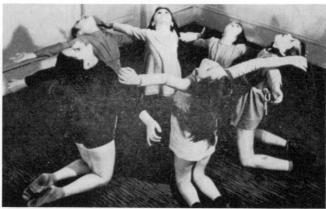

In our society, children are brought to a class to learn how to dance. How well they learn is seen from this illustration of a group ranging from four to ten year olds who were asked to make a circle and a backbend from a kneeling position. Children are capable of expressing extreme personal feeling in so simple a rite as this one.

We cannot with one swoop change a form of culture, but if we are aware of its trends and its deficiencies, we spread wide influence by *doing* what we believe. In the field of Dance, we face the problem of restoring the non-professional *role* of Dance. In the past few years, in the United States, the movement to revive traditional country folk dances for the city citizen, has been an important contribution in this direction. But there are other paths open in addition: the creation of dance activity, *in the dance studio*, not as a watered-down professional form, but as an unashamed, purely human activity existing in its own right, for specific needs, and thereby creating its own forms and techniques.

In our culture the Dance has been glamorized and professionalized and made almost sterile in the process, by being placed, along with music and painting, in museums, recital halls, cinema, radio, books, -- and now television -- and something ONLY to *see*, rather that to *do* or as something to do *lamely*.

As a result, the parent and child have taken a humble and demeaned place. Most parents to-day -- even the most progressive -- *apologize* when they register their children: "I know my child is no Pavlowa, or, "I know she's not very good at it, but she does love it so", etc. It is a sad comment on our society when the person feels he is overstepping his bounds when all he wants to do is to dance. Even worse than this, is the attitude expressed by the parents -- and their number is legion -- who say, "I know all this about rhythm, and body foundation work, and creative dance, but when will my child be ready to *really* dance?"

The teacher of vision who believes in the re-integration of theatre dance with life in its many ramifications, and of life with Dance, has an enormous task to-day of taking the Dance out of the *limitations* of the professional sphere and *releasing* it for *utilization*. And then what rich fields open up in education, in physical and mental therapy, in social adjustment, in the life of every day, whereby both the student and the profession have so much to gain.

This process of re-orientation is not easy since the dance teacher has the problem of finding peace for herself, for the child, and for the parent, between the two warring factors of the natural function of Dance and Western theatrical Dance; between the beautiful skilled movement of the artist of Dance -- truly most wondrous-- and the strangely bouncing body of the child as she twists and turns her little arms propelling herself through Space.

The next article in this series by Miss Evan will appear in the MAY, 1949 issue of DANCE Magazine.

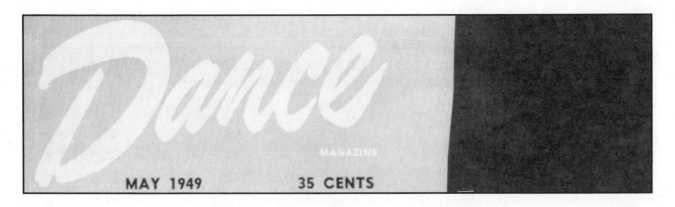
MAY 1949   35 CENTS

THE CHILD'S WORLD
Its relation to Dance Pedagogy
a series of articles by BLANCHE EVAN

Article III, in the MARCH issue, discussed the separation of generic dance from concert dance in western culture, and the specific problems caused thereby in dance technique for children. By "technique" I mean the transformation of functional body movement into skill with the purpose of extending the power of expression in dance.

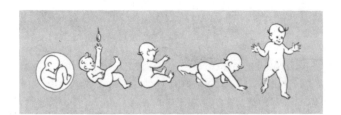

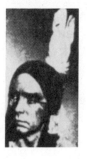

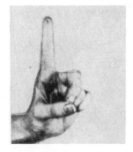

"Each infant renews the struggle". Photo: Dr. Mensendieck's "Functional Exercise".

Reginald Laugin wearing the "upright lone feather".

"I, boasting" from La Meri's "Gesture Language of the Hindu Dance".

The separate technique that fills an hour becomes meaningful only if it adds up to one meaningful whole. The teacher who believes in avoiding ready-made techniques and eclectic limitations is faced *essentially* with the needs of a *basic ideology* to guide the process of forming *new* technique, THIS IS AN ENORMOUS SUBJECT OPEN TO VAST INTERPRETATION, with numerous inter-related topics: over-all objective, subsidiary objectives that determine selection, philosophy of presentation, psychological implications in technical forms, inter-cultural aspects, sexual components, relation to specific environments, etc. It must be clearly understood, and accepted as a premise, that their ultimate formulation depends upon the teacher's philosophy or lack of one. There is no school of thought to adhere to. We are in the process of creating a technique.

Since we are creating this technique FOR the child of TO-DAY, it validity will greatly depend upon the relationship it establishes to the contemporary background in which the child lives.

In teaching Dance to American children, I have been repeatedly impressed with how foreign they have become to Dance as an *expressional* medium. I base my conclusions on the experience of having taught over a thousand children. The average American child considers it actually strange "to move" the body.

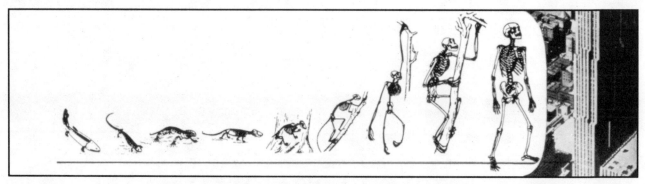

After efforts of millions of years to attain spinal verticality, Man has now created the City, which ignores the kinetic needs of his own body.

I found them lacking in natural co-ordination, and their musical response limited to foot patterings undifferentiated in dynamics and tempo. They had no directional sense of space and were unconscious of the rhythm of another person or a group. There was no grasp of dancing harmoniously in a circle or with a partner. It was shocking to watch them turn every dance formation into a game, more often to destroy, rather than to enjoy the unification of formation, or at best, to be oblivious to it; while every movement into space was used as an excuse for a competitive race. They were ignorant of "imagining" or "feeling" in terms of body movement. Their orientation to Dance seemed limited to a bundle of appropriated tricks.

Such was the little novice that rang the bell to register for dancing lessons. My immediate problem was to create for her a technique that would restore these values, because without them she couldn't dance. Without them, she couldn't even live too well, in my way of thinking. For self-confidence in body movement, rhythmic response, and social response were basic values essential in this as in any other time.

To help the child's body become an instrument of expression in dance, I found I had not only to start at the beginning, as a teacher expects to do, but I had to *undo*, even in the five year olds, a super-structure of barriers in which they had been encased. With every victory of transformation into a dancing body, shall I say, into a body now made ready for Dance. I was re-inforced in my contention that the children had been victim to the environmental characteristics of our particular culture.

Dance has always reflected the environment that produced it. The basic movement responses referred to above *are* known to untrained children of most other cultures but are seriously damaged in our own because our life apparently shuts them out.

Body movement, time and space have become mechanized for the child.

Mechanical life has virtually immobilized the body to minimum range.

Visual and auditory stimuli is over-abundant and ill chosen. The eye and ear are glutted by widespread use of radio, television, print and movies, whose furthest thought is the constructive development of the child.

The concept of "rugged individualism" with which the child is indoctrinated, clothes a kind of cut-throat rivalry, making of the child a very unsocial-minded creature.

The universal educational system in which the child lives one third of daily life, ignores the emotional life of the child and stifles the initiative, the concentration, the imagination.

There is such wide disparity between the "natural" child and the strivings and mores of our culture, as to over-tax the powers of adaptability of the child.

The child *lives* in this atmosphere, each factor of which has destructive effects upon her body movement. I am always in search of the forces at work that cause this destruction that I might better find the answers in terms of Dance activity; as I am also in search of the positive values of our culture to be utilized in Dance.

This is the meaning of my concept "Technique for the City". For although my work was developed to meet the needs of city children, the highly geared metropolis actually is an intensification and a concentrate of the the characteristics that distinguish our American culture, to which the child on the farm in North Dakota is subject as well as the child of the Big City.

I wish to state very emphatically that I am not an "anti-machine, anti-modern" romantic; but that this does not preclude a critical evaluation of our society.

The technical work for the child must include a specific plan for re-orientation to the values of body movement, individually and socially. It must re-establish the child's confidence in the body itself.

CONCEPT OF VERTICALITY

In our culture, the destruction of body confidence relates even to Man's basic anatomy--his vertical posture, which has taken him millions of years of spinal evolution to attain. *Each infant that is born has to renew that fight.* A synopsized version of the struggle takes place in the first two years of life, from the round foetal position, through sitting, crawling with the support of four appendages, *horizontally,* to finally assume "the human position." Animals *at birth* move in the exact vertebral position that they maintain through life, just as they rest in this position. The human being, to rest, has to change from the complete vertical to the complete horizontal, removing all weight from his base of support. His resistance to gravity is a strain. The interesting illustrations herewith briefly tell the story.

The upright spine is *not* fixed at the age when the child first stands, but is the *result of growth* that continues into young adulthood--growth of both bone and muscle. Even among controversial *systems of posture,* with which we are not here concerned, it is agreed that only by utilizing the mobility of the vertebrae and their related mechanisms can we *attain* their unified verticality. Only by muscular tonality can we *retain* it.

"The disuse atrophy of the bones seen in X-ray after wearing a cast even for a short time"--and this has been found also in hysteria paralysis--"is evidence enough of the necessity for activity and in normal children the development and hardness of the bones bears a direct relation to activity. As a corollary to this, the relative perfection of the posture therefore depends to a great extent upon activity. The posture of the normal child is a direct indication of his activity."

The fact that our children to-day grow taller than before may be due to the increased use of vitamins in diet that build bone. In this connection it is important to remember that *more than ever* we need muscles strong enough *to support the increased length* of bones, a poor ratio of development between the two.

"produces a comparative muscular weakness and consequent lack of co-ordination which is very evident and a causative factor in the adoption of postural attitudes and habits which often persist in the adult".

Science as yet has no "capsule substitute" for *harmonized bodily activity.*

The amount of resistance to torsal activity the child (and adult) manifests to-day in the Dance studio is inconceivable. They have lost the very idea of *muscular intensity* and of *joint manipu-*

lation, because of the dearth of body-action in daily experience. Even when supported by a thematic base, by an action-idea that in life could not be accomplished without spinal mobility, much discussion is necessary to create an imaginative response, and much prodding is then necessary to get the full participation of the body.

Last week, in desperation, I explained to a class of six year olds that children who plant and weed a garden have to bend down to the earth to do so; and those children whose fathers are fishermen, often bend forward and backward to help tug in a line, etc. But that in "city life"--mechanized life--we have little occasion to bend: "just to pick up a piece of paper", one of them said.

Themselves convinced, and therefore convincing to watch, for the first time in sixteen lessons, those children used their torsos thoroughly in action.

We are depriving the body of the activity need for building a strong spine. The lack of self-confidence that ensues is magnified because we continue to have a tenacious grip on the PSYCHOLOGICAL AND SOCIAL ATTRIBUTES with which we have invested Man's attainment of spinal verticality, and which have derived from it.

STANDARDS AND TABOOS

American Indian sign language for "Man" is the vertical index finger. Reginald Laubin tells us that this gesture must be done perfectly, because to the Indian the symbol means "The One Alone", since *only* Man is "upright", and therefore he alone can be proud. The same gesture is used by Australian tribes to mean "Myself", and in Hindu mudras, to mean "I, boasting". The American Indian also designates to the bravest man only, the headgear of the "upright lone feather," lesser braves being compelled to wear the feather at an angle diverging downward from the vertical line.

Many of our present standards and taboos are related to Man's achievement of spinal verticality: as a characteristic of superiority over the animal world; as an embodiment of his power to think, as a symbol for self-assurance, for courage, and when exaggerated, for aggressiveness.

Its opposite in posture, toward gravity, is equally significant, seeming to indicate insecurity, introversion, laziness, carelessness, and even defeat; plus the emotional intensification of downward direction in sorrow and retreat. We are aware of the enormously appealing satisfaction in forms of slouch, in passivity, and "rest" in death. We recognize the yearning for the return to the security of the round, foetal form, with its attendant relinquishment of independence; we are annoyed at the way children "lean" against walls and tables. We have contempt for a person who, as we say, "can't stand on his own two feet". At the other extreme, there is succinct social comment of superiority over other human beings, in the term, "regal carriage".

We are familiar also with the standards of sexual appeal related to posture: with the encasement of buttocks and bosom by American women today to lessen divergence from the straight, vertical line, with the "attractive" West Point upright physique, with the concept of the proud, unsubmissive woman who "holds herself like a Goddess", etc. and etc.

RELATED FIELDS

Following are quotes on the same subject from other fields:

"The words 'straighten up' imply traits of integrity and self-reliance".

"The substructure of ballet movement is a belief in the basic perpendicularity of the human being, man's most significant initial posture being his erect position on two legs"..."its elegance", (fundamental ballet position), "is the most simple, dignified assertion of man's spectacular possession of a power to stand on two feet, to balance his column of bone and flesh on a small flexible base..."

"...if generalizations were to be made about the causes of human diseases, it would be along the line of failure of accommodation to the erect posture..."

"...for defective posture entails habitually strained muscles and a lack of balance of the bones at the joints. A disturbed kinaesthesia and unbalance in the proprioceptive system follow closely in this trail..."

"Man may be said to live both horizontally and perpendicularly. His horizontal life consists of his social... relations; his perpendicular life is the direct flow of his blood and spirit."

At periodic intervals, Man has created concepts and structures in his own image: the placement of Heaven, directly upward: the architectural forms of totem poles, obelisks, (Egyptian for "ray of the sun"), pyramids, the Gothic spire, etc. We find vertical design accentuations on buildings of centuries past, as well as to-day, on the functional skyscraper, landmark of the City. Symbology only emphasizes the importance to himself, of Man's skeletal direction, upward.

Whether we wish to prepare the child's body to be the instrument of a form of Dance that exaggerates this verticality and seeming victory over gravity as does the Ballet in its extension to "the point"; or for a form of Dance which utilizes spinal deviations from verticality for their dramatic implications, as does the Modern Dance; or as instrument of the widest gamut of expression on a purely personal level, --a first requisite is a strong spine.

This precludes the active development of all its related mechanisms: the rib cage and pelvic girdle that extend horizontally from it; its appendages, arms and legs; the shoulder girdle; the head; the feet supporting the whole--each of them in need of technique not only in themselves, but because fundamentally *each* carries the responsibility of *building* a vertical spine.

In a society that pays these matters little heed, this becomes a focal point for Dance technique.

BIBLIOGRAPHY:
Dr. C. A. Aldrich—"Babies Are Human Beings"
Ruth Benedict—"Patterns of Culture"
Lincoln Kirstein—"Dance as Theatre"
W. C. Mackenzie—"Public Health Service of the U.S."
Dr. Bess Mensendieck—"Functional Excerise"
Dr. Phelps & R. J. Kiphuth—"The Diagnosis and treatment of Postural Defects"
E. Gladys Scott—"Analysis of Human Motion"
Mabel Ellsworth Todd—"The Thinking Body"

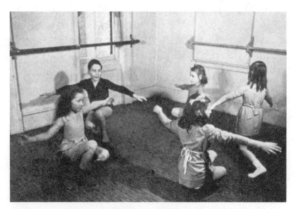

A spine-in-action is the basis for a straight spine.

Part II of "Technique for the City" will appear in the July issue.

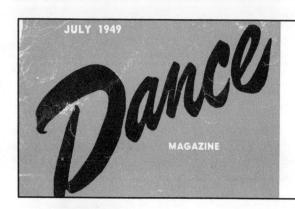

JULY 1949

Dance

MAGAZINE

35 CENTS

THE CHILD'S WORLD
It's Relation to Dance Pedagogy
a series of articles by BLANCHE EVAN

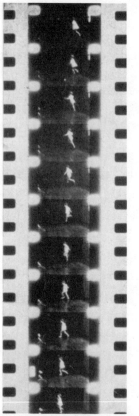

5-year old Jarmilla in "A Lesson in Rhythm". 16 mm. film by Fred Fehl. Script by Blanche Evan.

ARTICLE V
Technique for the City

PART II: HEART-BEAT

Part I of "Technique for the City", May issue, pointed out that dance technique for the modern child "must include a specific plan for re-orientation to the values of body movement, individually and socially".

It also stated that the strength of the child's body as an instrument of Dance will depend in large measure on the range and intensity of the *movement* of its spinal structure and related mechanisms.

We must, almost in the same breath, speak of *rhythm*, without which movement is chaos.

The rhythm of sound, action, sight, and feeling, etc., are inter-related. The rhythm of the waves is co-ordinated with the sound the waves produce. The rhythm of a lullaby is usually associated with the feeling of rocking, and of being rocked by one who loves you. Rhythm of action would seem to be the union of dynamics and tempo, space direction and content, characterized essentially by periodicity.

The movement of any good dancer, regardless of style or type, is rhythmic. All the joints and muscles move in relation to each other, subject to the rhythm content of the whole. In a poor dancer, the joints seem to move without regard for any unified objective. The average child to-day in the Dance class moves very *unrhythmically*, moves the *same* way to *different* music, and is insensitive to the rhythm of another individual or group. The older the children, the less rhythmic they are. Four year olds learn to march in time more easily than children of five.

Yet infants act rhythmically from the moment they are born. They also respond to rhythmic sound. A lullaby induces sleep; and at the age of six to nine months, children beat perfect time to music.

Apparently instinctive rhythm-for-action is lost unless given an opportunity for continued practise. *In our society* there is little chance for its survival without specialized training, because mechanized life deprives the child of rhythmic experience. The child in natural surroundings is exposed to nature's *environmental rhythms*--the waving wheat in the wind, for instance. She is often an integral part of the *rhythmic work* of production, of planting and gathering, etc. The city child is not involved with the rhythms of growing things. She "pays money" for an impersonal object already grown, even cooked, frozen and tinned.

Rhythmic play for the city child is also conditioned by mechanical equipment.

The very contact of *the child's foot* on turf and sand produces rhythmic spring and resilience; whereas in the city, the child's *walking experience*

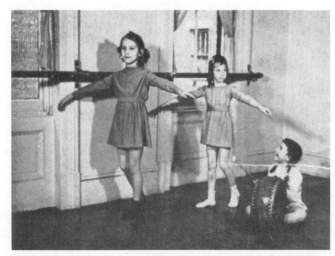
Children learn to adjust to each other's rhythms.

takes place in a leather sole on lifeless cement; "the step" becoming a succession of horizontal blurred progression in space. Our children lose the vitality of the foot very early in life. Yet resilient rhythmicity of the foot step is the very basis of locomotion in dance.

The city child not only lacks personal rhythmic experience. She is also thrust headlong into the city atmosphere of speed, frenzy, acceleration and the city chaos of space, action, sight and sound. Skyscrapers stand squeezed between two story buildings and vice versa. Electric lights are multicolored and glare and blink from every level. Clamorous din blares out from a multiplicity of sources. A child takes a walk in the street through the roar of traffic, a ride in the subway train after its onrushing approach into the station, the tumult of the crowds everywhere, a quick lift in the elevator. Then inside the house, filled with the confusion of radio programs,--where *music is merely a background* for family conversation, household chores, reading, quarreling, vacuum cleaning, with advertising jargon and commercials interspersed. At the end of the hectic day, cohorts of canned story tellers oozing out sentimentalities and horrendous tales, supplant the "old-fashioned" soothing rhythm of a sleeping song and comforting peace rhythm of the bed-time story.

We are familiar with all of this; but we must also understand that *our children are affected* by it. The average child *cannot, by herself*, build a rhythmic body. Yet obviously, she can't dance without one. Therefore,--and though this may not have been necessary in the nineteenth century, TO-DAY the child's dance technique must include *specific training in Rhythm.*

The teacher has to learn to understand the *rhythm of children*, so vastly different from the adults'. In addition, *each child* has a rhythm of her own, expressive of her total personality. Of prime importance in the Technique of Rhythm I have developed for children, from three years upward, is the *relation* of Rhythm to Age, Personality, the Group, and the Progression of Technical Skill; also the *integration* of kinaesthetic rhythm with content, and the *response* of rhythm to auditory and visual stimuli.

PERIODICITY

Everyone is born with rhythm. To "teach" it resolves itself essentially into how to RESTORE the child's *instinctive* rhythm. Work in temporal rhythm should precede spatial rhythm.

The first task is to bridge the gap for the child between the chaotic sound of her environment and the basic element of rhythm, its periodicity. The very idea of periodicity suggests order and the kind of *security that derives from regularity*. It is the antitheses of the anxiety that accompanies confusion.

Isolating the rhythmic beat is the most direct means to re-establish periodicity. We cannot use music for this too well, because first we must help the child divest herself of the mass of undifferentiated music she has been exposed to. Our children have to learn to respect music as something *to select* and *to listen to* before they can respond rhythmically to it. We can get down to its rhythmic core, by stripping music of both melody and harmony, leaving pulse beat itself.

In this work, I have found the use of the drum and tambourine to be the shortest route to achieving rhythmic results. The drum keeps a constant pitch, and even in its use of restricted steady beat, its dynamic range is wide. This is of special value, since the use of the periodic beat becomes more meaningful with dynamic variation.

We may play a marked, regular beat for a child, but we cannot be sure she *hears it regularity,* or that she can *transpose* it to body action. Therefore, I have the child herself play a drum or tambourine to establish, from the outset, "audio-kinesthesia",--if I may coin the word,--"hearing-doing". The child from the first this *associates* the *sound-beat with her own body action.* She is guided by the tempo of my louder drum. When the beat is firmly established, the child is asked to cease her playing. She is able to transfer *her* sound association to the sound of the *teacher's* drum, while *retaining her rhythmic action*: of arms, of body; then, foot locomotion, and last of all, body action through space.

For the child, the beat should be not only *steady* in tempo, but played at a rate *set at the general level of children.* For instance the tempo of an arm swing for a four year old child should be much faster than for a child of eight, though it should be much slower than the rate of gallop for the same four year old. By setting a *functional* rate in the basic training of the child, she comes to regard rhythm not as "keeping time", but as a pulse to which she is able to respond with her *whole* self.

A WORD ABOUT THE DRUM

The drum has a strange power, *when used with a plan,* to develop the rhythmic ability where none seems manifest. It has been used as a focus of rhythm in the life and dance of cultures all over the world; but I was interested to discover its fascination for the modern child, who can sit alone for twenty minutes at a time, perfectly happy, playing,--not banging--the drum, sometimes with a never varying beat.

Two summers ago, in a Course of Dance Pedagogy I gave to a group of Negro public school teachers at North Carolina College of Durham, I asked students why they thought the drum was such a perfect medium for rhythmic training. I quote from one of the papers presented:

"Before we make the first move toward dancing let us find an instrument that will aid us in rhythm and will be most naturally in tune with our bodies. Think of all the organs in the body. Which, if it should stop its rhythmic motions, would effect your life most? Surely, the heart. We find that the drum is almost exactly like the tone of the heart beat. This beat is common to us all."

I have found no explanation so inclusive of the practical, social and psychological implications of the rhythmic beat. It even relates to many findings in psychology: e.g., "the heart often serves as a time keeper and as a pace-maker".

There are many technical transitions and developments within the fundamental sphere which I cannot describe here: for instance, the transition from drum to music. Also, the children's use of the subdivided beat and its multiples. But this comes naturally in the *process* and *progress* of becoming *more* rhythmic. NUMBERS SHOULD NEVER BE USED in fundamental rhythmic training. Counting 1,2,3 has *arithmetic*, not *rhythmic* association for the child. Meter: 3/4, 2/4, time, etc, also should not be introduced as such until the child has developed rhythmicity. If she can determine the *main* pulse beat, her rhythmic response will *logically* expand into a measure and a phrase.

Blanche was learning from children rather than "teaching"

The span of periodicity grows with experience. The child becomes conscious of the pulse beat in sound accompaniment of different tempi. This helps her to cope with the technical problems involved in executing action at a tempo slower or faster than the functional tempo of a particular movement. Guided by the pulse beat, she responds rhythmically to different meter, different timbre and dynamics, whether in percussion or music, and so her improvisations begin to take on rhythmic form

To demonstrate how *unmechanical* and how *related to life* the building of periodicity can be: in the five to seven year old group, I played a soft cymbal in a regular beat. When I found that a number of children were not responding, I asked what the sound reminded them of. The responses *in words* were: "the flapping wings of a bird", "church bell", "soft wind", etc. It wasn't long before the room was filled with rhythmic improvisation.

The rhythmic sense becomes so well developed that the child eventually improvises, rhythmically, in silence.

Having laid the *foundation* in temporal rhythm, it is easier to tackle the technical problems of periodicity of space rhythm, and of the rhythm of content.

TEMPO AND RHYTHM

TO BUILD the child's rhythm, it is necessary for the teacher to have an accuracy of tempo to a metronomic degree. If the teacher lacks this accuracy, the rhythm of the child's movement is in conflict with the auditory stimulus, producing non-rhythmic activity. If the teacher is not able to control her tempo, she should avoid the use of percussion for precise rhythm work, but use, instead, the simplest kinds of music played on a machine where tempo is controlled for her.

It is important to reiterate, however, that tempo, though basic, is only one element in rhythm, and that divested of dynamics, and content, it becomes a cold, objective thing. I have seen many children "dancing" in perfect time, but lifelessly, without the dynamic life of rhythm. The building of dynamic sensitivity should proceed along with periodicity, but it requires other considerations. For instance, emotion expresses itself rhythmically even though, it is often difficult and, for expressional purposes, unnecessary, to analyze its periodic span.

Because rhythm is an expression of the total personality, it is most important that the work in periodicity always include opportunities for the child to determine her own rhythm for movement.

Rhythm is first of all a functional arrangement in all of nature.

Christopher Caudwell, in his study of poetry, has said very beautifully: "Rhythm shouts aloud the dumb processes of the body's secret life."

Recently, a psychiatrist brought to my attention the attempts made in his own field to understand the phenomenon of rhythm. Only one of a dozen authors mentions Dance! On the other hand, Dance has neglected the vast *psychological* importance and implications of rhythm to children.

These quotes from psychiatric writings are relevant:

"...the foetus is constantly exposed to a variety of rhythmic experiences, the most prominent of which is the aortic pulse...It is conceivable that during times of stress or tension the infant could be, through rhythmic body activity attempting to recreate the conditions of the period of its life in which it had its greatest security."

"Muscular activity, both voluntary and involuntary, has a strong tendency to be periodic...and the rhythms of several activities, e.g., pulse, respiration, stepping,...are usually in accord."

"...there is no rhythmic experience which is limited to one form of sensation. Rhythmic experience is a grouping of auditory, kinesthetic, tactual and visual stimuli. These are inter-related, and dependent on each other."

Let the children speak for themselves. Recently I said to my eleven year old class: "We do so much work here in rhythm--please write down what it means to you". Above are excerpts in photostat:

The last is perhaps the most significant. By crossing out and rewriting, this child said in her own way that:

To re-build rhythm means to develop a RHYTHMIC CONSCIOUSNESS that will act as the BASIS for rhythmic co-ordination of movement to external stimuli.

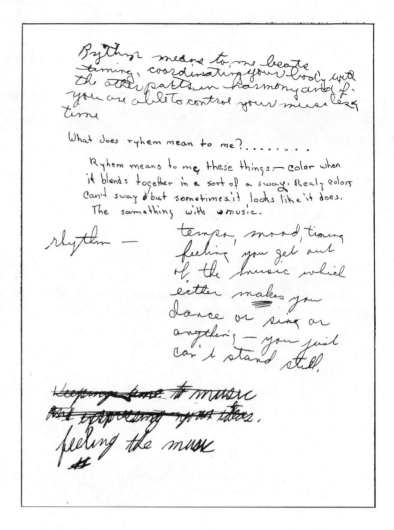

Since the child of "the City" is denied identification with rhythm, in the Dance class we must dig into the realm where instinctive rhythm itself lies dormant.

Part III of "Technique for the City" will appear in the October issue.

NOVEMBER 1949

Dance
MAGAZINE

35 CENTS

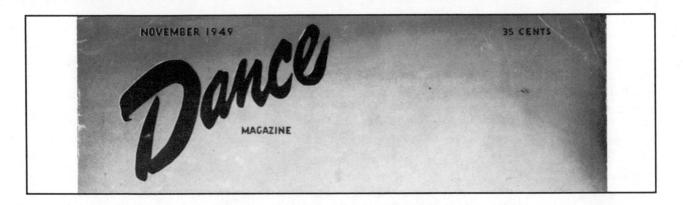

THE CHILD'S WORLD
Its Relation to Dance Pedagogy
a series of articles by BLANCHE EVAN

ARTICLE VI
Technique for the city

PART III — RHYTHM OF SHARING

The child of "the City" essentially is a lonely child. The many efforts made to-day to involve the child in "group activity" is uniquely characteristic of our time, and in tacit recognition of the truth that the modern child is isolated from the group.

Our society does not integrate the child in social living, as do less mechanized cultures. For instance, in most parts of the world, we see the children directly engaged in the work rhythms that sustain life. Where we cannot directly observe, work songs relate to us the work of the fields, the sea, the guilds: the work of swinging the sharp blade of the scythe around, in perfect timing with one's neighbor; of coordinating with others in the horizontal pull of a boat filled with the evening's catch; of exerting the intensity needed to tame the young colt, and to prod the oxen to labor, etc.

These work rhythms involve the total human being. They often require interchangeable action with at least one other person, and an intimate knowledge of the forces of nature. The whole body performs as a unit in action that demands a functional intensity and a sharpened space-time unified rhythm. The objective of the whole work is never lost, but is manifest in the moment-to-moment process of the work.

The Occupational Fiestas and many of the Community Dances, *in which the children and adults jointly participate*, revolve around the Work Theme. For example, the dances: "PLANTING RICE" -- Philippine Islands; "SCHUHPLATTER", (SHOE CLAPPING), -- Austria; "BEAN SETTING" -- England; "DEBNARSKEY", (HOOP MAKERS), -- Germany; "AUGONELI", (POPPY PLANTING), -- Lithuania, etc.

The child grows up sharing both work and play with adults and with other children equally involved. In these cultures, *the child is needed* in community life. She maintains a *functional* role in the Social Rhythm of her environment.

In large sections of modern life, the child does not contribute to the work rhythm of her time. Work is

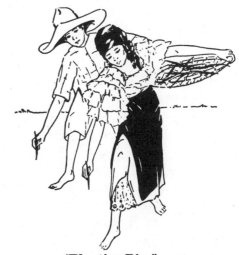

"Planting Rice"
OCCUPATIONAL dance of the Philippine Islands.

removed from the home, and from the life of the family, except in its economic import. The adult members of the household, after pursuing their separate work of the day, meet with the child, when they do, at the hurried supper table. Every effort is made to delay the time when the child will have to participate in work.

Let us examine the rhythm of this work.

WORK RHYTHM OF "THE CITY"

THE CITY" (mechanized life) contains multitudinous perfect rhythms of *inanimate* machines. The machine typifies most kinds of work in "the city", including that of the office worker. The division of labor compels the worker to move in a circumscribed sphere. He does not feel the stimulus of contributing to the final product. The action in most cases is repetitive, subject to the mute demands of the machine, and to the employer's standard of efficiency. As mechanization increases, there is less and less involvement of the total human being with the machine. In our present Economic nexus, -- I speak of America -- when the worker permits himself to become "totally" involved, chaos results -- as Charlie Chaplin so magnificently revealed in his film "MODERN TIMES". Chaos results because maximum efficiency in our machine production depends more and more upon the total IMMOBILITY of the human being, and upon his mastery of isolating, from the rest of himself, those parts of his body and his mind necessary in running the machine.

THE RHYTHM OF THIS WORK IS CHARACTERIZED BY *DETACHMENT* FROM THE VERY WORK RHYTHM THAT CONSUMES ONE THIRD OF DAILY LIFE. Our society has misused the machine, making it the antagonist to a good social life.

DANCE RHYTHM OF "THE CITY"

The most typical dance of the city, Jazz, mirrors, as true Dance always does, the life of the time -- in this case, segregation from the group. Jazz admits only two people, steering a path on a mobbed dance floor, much like a private automobile in dense traffic.

The mass rhythm is a sum total of organized nervous isolation.

Our professional corps de ballets also reflect this status. *The Ballet companies in America are notoriously lacking in group co-ordination.* The modern dance groups are usually whipped into unity by the dominating personality of the choreographer. The most perfect dancing corps -- and widely admired -- is that of the sterile Rockettes of Radio City; it makes no pretense at being anything more than a human version of detached mechanization, typical rhythm of the society that produced it.

NECESSITY OF SHARING

Yet to-day, life is more inter-dependent than ever before. In its social context, the world becomes smaller each day, despite the blindness of men who pretend they can rule it otherwise, -- while our child grows up either ignorant of social living or psychologically hostile to it. Denied enlargement of rhythm as a sharing experience in work actions of daily living, denied rhythmic dance and song and play that reflect and complement it, lacking rhythms called forth by direct contact with nature, separated in most ways from the adult world, -- for this modern child there is no *rhythm of the group*.

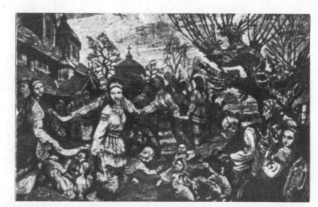

Holiday in early 19th century Russia — participation by children in group dancing

In this set-up, *can* we produce for the child an UNARTIFICIAL social group rhythm, replacing isolation with integration? Is it possible to form a connecting link between the rhythms of other cultures and the radically different rhythm of the child's own environment of to-day? Can we counteract the anti-social propaganda *directed* to the modern child?

It would be dangerous to assume that any one activity could solve a problem which is inherent in the structure of present society itself. However, we must

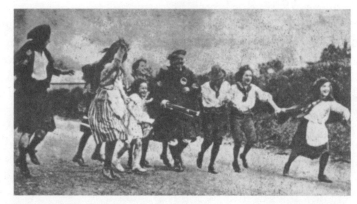

"Children and adults jointly participate..." festival in Ireland.

at least assume the responsibility that IN EACH OF THE CHILD'S ACTIVITIES, WE DEVELOP THE MEANS *APPROPRIATE TO THAT ACTIVITY*, TO INITIATE A *SOCIAL RHYTHM* AS *PROFOUND* AS CAN BE DERIVED FROM THE MEDIUM AT HAND.

THE FIELD OF DANCE IS RICH AS A SOURCE FOR RHYTHMS OF SHARING.

THE COMMON DENOMINATOR

In a class of children, we must find an orbit to which the rays of many disparate personalities will be drawn. We must find *a common denominator*.

"Rhythm puts people...in touch with each other . . . physiologically and emotionally . . . when each retires into his body and shares the same . . . elemental beat." (Caudwell) This has been known throughout Time, but has been forgotten in the pursuit of arduous virtuosity in the Dance of Spectacle.

The marked periodicity of rhythm is the base for individual restoration of rhythm (see Article V, July issue), and for group unification as well. The *rhythmic beat* has universal appeal, and gathers response regardless of age, personality, sex, character, environment, etc. It can be a tremendous force in group solidification. In Dance, it is a basic binder for many diverse forms of group rhythm.

The individual child's newly organized sense of rhythm, colored by her characteristic personality rhythm, *fuse* to-gether with that group rhythm typical of her general age level, constituting the process of *levelling* without which there can be no group rhythm.

Sharing the rhythmic beat takes many forms; the children *play in unison*, the basic rhythms -- basic, but none the less exciting. They *share anticipation* in the dynamic swells of rhythms and *harmonious group movement* to quiet accompaniment. They execute simple technique *with a partner* or more, set at the *group functional rate*. They dance in *duets and trios and groups*, the *rhythms of work* of the past and present, and *those of familiar play*. they *create together social rhythms of content* that appeal to the particular group at the particular time. They *dance together* to the delightful *beat of the ethnic music of the world*.

CONTEMPORARY IMAGES

I remember the period of "machine dances" in early modern dance. They were always scorned by the seers and peers, perhaps because they were in a stage of naturalism rather that of insight. Nonetheless, just as the children of Lithuania do their dance, "Augoneli", -- "Poppy Planting", I feel it is appropriate to utilize contemporary images of our children, *to awaken them to the social import of the rhythm of their time*.

The realistic rhythm of the machine is clear-cut and precise, and can be helpful in building clear periodicity in group action. Machine images can be used as the basis of creative group improvisation, and of simple choreographic studies. The child's range of fantasy can thus be widened to include the contemporary scene. For instance, last season, the nine year old group automatically chose a traditional fairy tale as the improvisational theme of the lesson. Through detailed discussion, leading from the bus that took them to school each day, back to the spokes of the first wooden wheels, they formulated a theme which so fascinated them that they spent many hours in the creation of a finished dance. The theme was: "A lady 2000 years from now wants to know what our times were like. She pressed a magic button and saw":--a complex choreographic arrangement entitled "WHEELS", consisting of shifting numbers of people working to-gether in circles and squares, weaving about and supine on the floor, -- a truly intriguing group dance, imaginative and integrated, created by the children, but made possible only by their new insight into their environment.

RHYTHMS OF OCCUPATION

The re-enactment of all work themes of past and present, realistically and imaginatively, make excellent material for rhythms of sharing. The best starting point, I have found, is the *functional rhythm* of the work theme. There are available to-day numerous record albums that have re-captured an authentic spirit of the work songs of both the past and present: old English Sea Chanties, modern Soviet Union harvest songs, traditional American songs of the work on the levees and railroad, cotton picking songs of the South, etc. There are also delicate work songs: of basket weaving in the Carribean, and the potter's wheel in India. There are folk songs strummed on guitars, authentic sound recordings, and a variety of more abstract music, by our foremost modern composers, that has been based on rhythms of occupation.

With the rhythm of work so alien to the modern child, creative stimulation on the part of the teacher is an essential. It can take many forms including the use of illustrative material, and comparison, in terms of dance and music, among the rhythms of different cultures.

THE FARANDOLE

This article has confined itself to the Social Rhythms of Work and their application in the Dance studio. Lack of space prevents discussion of other kinds of Rhythms of Sharing to be utilized in Dance: for instance, rhythms of play and rhythms of Nature. THE EFFECTIVENESS OF THE MATERIAL DEPENDS IN GREAT MEASURE UPON *YOUR OBJECTIVE* IN THE USE OF IT.

Folk dance is group dance in elemental and enduring form. It is not necessary to teach authentic folk dances. The use of folk patterns known the world over: dancing in a circle, in squares and lines, turning under a partner's arm, etc., -- these forms are directly social, and delight children of any age.

The Farandole form is one of the most popular with the children. The group forms a chain, and is led by each child in turn, in a step of her own choosing. The children love it -- because, in its own way, it takes cognizance of the need to balance individual striving with group function.

EACH AGE GROUP REQUIRES ITS OWN TECHNIQUES IN BUILDING RHYTHMS OF SHARING. In all of them it is important to provide the individual child with plenty of opportunity to express her own rhythm. This is necessary to balance the strain of group rhythm which she is experiencing, and because, *the richest social rhythm is achieved by the contributions of highly developed individuals.*

In a future article, I will discuss pedagogical techniques for achieving this balance. Article VII will appear in the January, 1950 issue.

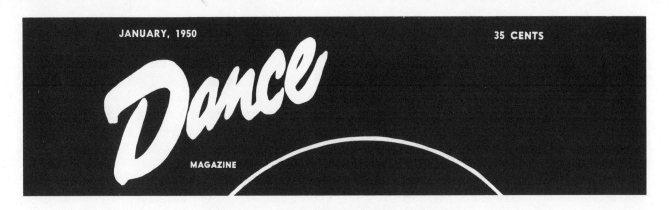
JANUARY, 1950   35 CENTS

Dance

MAGAZINE

Who is EVERYBODY?

the 3 to 5 year old in dancing class
by Blanche Evan

article VII of the series
"THE CHILD'S WORLD"

We were sitting in a circle on the floor: a group of ten children, three to five years old. "Everybody please do this", I requested, as I demonstrated a movement. No one moved. "Who is everybody?" I asked. No one answered. Who IS Everybody?" I questioned. "ME,...and her, and her, and her,..." a three and a half year old replied, pointing with precision to each and every child in turn.

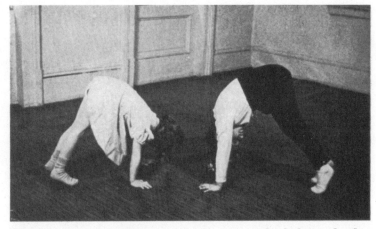

"The 3 to 5 year old group can learn a great deal about rhythm and functional exercises .. "

The pronouns "me" and "I" can be heard fifty times in a hours' class: "Watch *me*", *I* did it better than she did it", etc. There seem to be specific devices known to childhood to direct attention to the "me": one child will pull a circle to pieces, or form a little gang, another will do any exercise other than the one you've designated, another will refuse to do anything at all. Whereas in a five to seven year old group, you may find two out of fifteen behaving in this manner, in the three to five group, the behavior described is typical of many.

In this age group, the world starts with "Me" and centers around "Me". At one extreme we have the child who shouts "Me *first*" as she pushes others out of her way, and at the other, the child who, in learning about "Us" and "All together", is so struck with the idea, that she repeatedly asks, "Me too? Me too?"

Who is this little "me"? In a lesson in basic contrasts, I asked the four year olds to do "a big strong dance"; and to stimulate response, I posed the question, "Whom do you know who is big and strong?"--thinking, myself, in terms of Giants, Policemen, Daddys, etc.--when the tiniest, timidest child rang out her answer "ME". For a year, this child had spent much of her class time withdrawn, sucking her thumb. At this point, she stepped forth into a strong improvisation, charged with energy and rhythmic intensity.

The child at this age changes continually depending on the influences she is exposed to. She is a little person trying desperately to find her place in the world, adapting, and adopting, different attitudes and behaviors, to accomplish the task. The same child who is shy in the presence of a group, may be seemingly free at home; the disrupter in your class may be a "model" child at home or in a group differently constituted from yours. Furthermore, although the child's world is minute in perspective, potentially she is capable of as yet undefined ability.

The "Me" that presents itself, should be exposed to every constructive stimulus. If we teach the child on the level of the surface "me", we are guilty of encouraging the child's negative qualities and attitudes, at a time when, with comparative ease, they can be redirected to the positive. Furthermore, if you accept the "me world: as ultimate, you will have to pare down the wide field of Dance to a minute, individualistic level. You will have to distort your subject. Knowledge is a social entity. The child can become a recipient of knowledge if her potentials are externalized and her little world broadened. Exposed to a well organized group, the little child eventually realizes that others of her age share her fears, and her joys, her inadequacies and her prowess. The tiny mite who did the "big, strong dance" released a flow of self-confident movement among her classmates.

The *major pedagogic problem* in this age group of three to five years is to establish a positive social relation that ties together children, teacher, and the work at hand, changing the center of attention from a little dot in a big world, to a world just the right size.

METHODS

Simple group formations offer one means of establishing such a relation. The circle, holding hands, is the most effective and easiest "Us" to form. It is secure, everybody can see everybody all at once, and the "Me" belongs. The circle form is much easier to grasp than a line form, in which the "Me" sees no reason for retaining a set place in line. However, giving each child a chance to "lead" the line is a good device. It satisfies those who *want* to lead. Those who don't want to follow, do so knowing they will have a chance to lead. those who are afraid to do most things alone, seem always to enjoy leading a line in a simple march.

Dancing with one other person, unless she is your special friend or cousin, is much harder than dancing in a circle. One "ME" faces another "ME", eye to eye, and either complete ecstasy results, or if one dominates the other, both usually end up on the floor in a tumble. One little four year old manoeuvred a very complex arrangement with her "partner" in which both hands were crossed with those of the subjected one, in such a way as to necessitate the little tyrant dancing in front of the other, all the time. She used the same device when we changed partners.

Dancing with one other, or with a group in circles, lines, etc., are choreographic forms utilized in this age group *primarily for their social implication*. A four year old summarized our lesson on partners with this definition: "It means to take someone's hand", she said. What a lovely image.

There are diverse pedagogic means for widening the child's horizon to "Us": waiting a turn becomes acceptable only if the child is repeatedly assured by word and action that no one in class is ever deprived of her turn; watching each other, becoming aware that each has a contribution to make; sometimes copying a partner, sometimes leading; changing partners, as in "calling", folk dance style; clapping hands while resting, for the part of the group that is dancing; thematic material that builds good relationships, etc.

DISCIPLINE

Discipline should be based on how to help the child develop her best potentialities *and* function well with the group.

Finding herself in a sympathetic atmosphere, a child may drop many of the devices and defenses she has built up in other situations. For instance, if she feels very much at ease in your class, and if she has been reminded too often by other adults to "be a big girl", she may revert to crawling in the class room. Let her crawl for a while. Another will join her, and half the class may soon be on all fours. If we understand this aberration as a reversion to infancy, disciplinary measures, as such, will only mean to the child that it is more wrong to feel like a baby than to fake being a big girl. Rather than urge or command the child to cease, try to re-establish interest: convert the crawling to an animal study that involves technical problems, choose a baby theme for emotional release, or present a dance situation in contrast to the former part of the lesson. Try to understand their motivations for their behavior, and handle your disciplinary problems in relation to them, as much as possible. Don't be a martyr of patience. Only your understanding coupled with a desire to help will hold up as a source of tolerance and patience.

Unless psychologically ill, the disruptive child can be brought around through kindly methods: sometimes giving her added responsibility in the group is most effective. In most age groups, "to miss a turn is severe punishment. The issue is not primarily to "keep order" in class, but to convince our children that with order we can learn to dance--without it, we cannot. "Punishment", therefore, should never be meted out without a simple explanation to both the culprit and the class.

Be careful of over-talking. Most of what adults say does not relate to the child's experience and so succeeds only in separating teacher from child. Choose your words. I once heard a teacher say: "Let's get rid of our drums" instead of "Let's put them away:. On the other hand, learn the child's language: "Do you know what I have home?" a three year old asked me. "No, what?" "A big run", she said. Explain things, but don't argue with children on a level of adult logic. One little girl for a whole year referred to "her sister", though she knew, I knew, the child referred to was a friend, and that she had no sister at all.

Let the child sometimes use the natural abstract sounds she emits as she dances. Don't be harsh about stopping her Joycian flow of words. Re-direct her interest, intensify it in terms of dance, and she will cease the stream of talk and sound.

The child wants to experiment in movement. Give her this opportunity. Help her to discover herself, through Dance. There are many things she is experiencing in your classroom, for the very *first* time in her life.

AFRAID

We need a great deal of gentleness in the classroom. One unsocial child may be aggressive, another may retreat, another may cry, and the three may act from a single base--of fear. Let the teacher realize the enormous FEAR of our children. Some fears are open. Said Patsy: "I want to do a tiger dance, it won't be a real tiger, will it, because I'm afraid of tigers". Some fears are hidden. A very alert five year old refused to participate in a swing we were doing, a swing that evolved from the children's delight in monkeys. She said "no"--she had never seen a monkey. This did not seem possible to me. In discussing it with the mother, the mother said, "Of course, she has seen lots of monkeys--but she used to be terribly afraid of them. I thought she had gotten over it."

Children are very sensitive to their real or imagined physical inferiorities. In addition, most children have unfortunately been made ashamed of inability or failure, and rather than say, "I can't", a child will say, "I don't want to". She usually wants very much to "hop on one leg" or "lift way up", etc.; and usually, if you suggest doing it with her, the little shadow of sulkiness (fear) on her face changes to tentative hope, and eventually to the eagerness of participation.

The child should never be forced. With help and encouragement, most children are convinced that by doing, progress is made, and thereby fear lessened. The value of this positive attitude to physical effort, with its resultant gain in body stability and in over-all self-confidence, cannot be over-emphasized. It is a prerequisite to the learning of Dance.

THE DANCE

In addition to all the hidden fears and aggressions with which our children are burdened when they come to class, we place them in an untenable situation--in an empty room, with no playground equipment, no toys, *and no precedent in experience*, and we expect them to "learn dancing". Either they have never seen any, or they have seen the commercial, routine television type. Most of them have never seen their parents dance--the closest source of suggestion. And not knowing what it is all about, the uninhibited children begin to shout, and roll, and pull, and run around the big, empty room, while the scared ones get as far away from the emptiness as they can and crouch against the wall. In desperation, the teacher resorts to "imitating" a bunny or a bird and lets it go at that.

Throughout this article, I have very consciously used the word "dance" because a three year old, if registered in your class, is there to learn dancing, or, shall we say, to be exposed, under direction, to those elements of the Dance that can contribute to her whole development. The purpose is neither to "have fun" in the sense of playground, nursery games, etc., nor to have a formalised approach unsuitable for such a young child.

A three to five year old can learn a great deal about basic Rhythm. She can profit by functional exercise to strengthen muscles of the foot, stomach, shoulders, etc. She can be taught dynamic control of the body in movement and she can be directed to the enjoyment of participation in the social aspects of Dance. She can be helped enormously to gain security in the use of her body, and to experience an open response to inner feeling, and to the stimulus of sound. The kind of technical skill that is part of Dance is unique, and is not duplicated in games and sports. The child can also be stimulated in terms of imagination and creativity. In other words, *this youngest group can be taught Dance*, if we teach it, both in content and in presentation *with regard for the child's age.*

If we claim to be teachers of Dance, we will solve the pedagogic problems of teaching three to five year olds, *not by avoiding Dance*, but by *drawing out that part of Dance* that can contribute to the development of the total personality of a three to five year old.

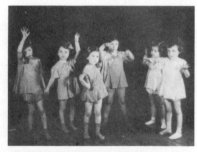

Improvising: What do they feel?

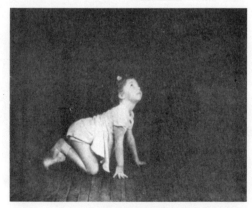

Improvising.

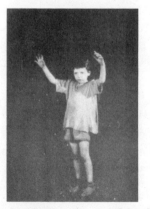

". . . fear clouds the face of this child . . ."

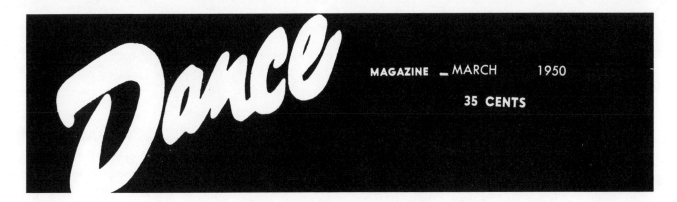

MAGAZINE — MARCH   1950

35 CENTS

"I am the SUN"
article VIII of the series:
THE CHILD'S WORLD
Its Relation to Dance Pedagogy
by Blanche Evan

"I WANT TO BE A PUPPET" says a 7 year old in class, "with one arm broken and one arm good". "With or without music?" is my only comment.

It is not by chance this child expresses herself so freely, after many weeks of tense, self-conscious behavior. She is proof again that creativity is often hidden; that resistance may be the cause of seeming barrenness, and that there are manifold ways of breaking through resistance; that creativity should be a part of every learning, and that for those who are not naturally gifted, there are distinct methods employable to stimulate the imagination in terms of Dance.

THE EMPTY SHELL

The idea of limiting class activity to "technique", *especially* for the one hour a week student, always seemed to me a vulgarization of Dance. After all, the most significant contribution of the new dance had been the resurgence of personalized experience in movement with its resultant re-assertion of individuality in form. I believe the dance lesson carried with it the responsibility of keeping this alive. This went hand in hand with my conviction that the technique should be physiological, functional, and impersonal, *not* stylized and dramatic. The skillful body free of mannerism would be the most adequate channel for individual creativity.

To limit teaching to technique and choreography, left a wide gap, for between the two there was imagination, without which both technique and choreography were an emptied shell -- a display. One could recognize the presence of creativity and point out the lack of it, but there were no methods at hand to help the average or repressed student to develop quality in Dance, personal style, and creative form: nor was there any suitable repertoire of dances, outside of folk and ethnic material, for interpretative practice. When given the opportunity to "dance", many students sat, frozen with fear. Some would dance *with* others, but not alone. Others would dance alone at home, but not in the presence of class mates. The students rarely felt, and moved with, that absorption in movement that distinguishes true Dance from superficial moving about.

Originality seemed a burden. Most preferred to be taught "a set dance"; but I went to the opposite pole, and chose improvisation as the main source for their creative work; improvisation: the spontaneous coming out of self into the realm of Dance, body, mind, and spirit unified and at the complete service of one's theme, regardless of the significance and duration of that theme.

Improvisation had always been for me a natural experience; but to develop methods, feeling had to be substantiated with analysis.

PROCEDURES

Improvisation is the spontaneous creation of form. Form and content ideally are one. Dance improvisation is the complete welding of yourself, as you are at the moment, with your theme, in terms of Dance. The beginning is the moment of merging; development proceeds, climax is achieved, and there is only one right moment for the end, when the theme, as it relates to you, has spun out its course. The child instinctively knows this, "I am finished" she says, though the music may not have terminated; or, the look of slight distress, if accompaniment ceases before she is through. I remember a six year old who improvised to a recording seven successive times before she was "finished".

Improvisation implies absorption, concentration and honesty. Not just to move about, nor to try to create, nor to imitate. Improvisation is dependent on an over-all state of receptivity which permits a free flowing stream of associative content, externalized into action. Self-consciousness is replaced with identification with your theme. Improvisation is the thread that winds and weaves, that binds and connects, that is the conductor for the whole self. At the point of action, it is the summation of your past and present. It is also the arbiter between reality and fantasy. "Even if I dance about lightness of snow in the night, I am still human doing it" a twelve year old explains.

In the process of breaking down creative activity, experimenting with means, and observing student reactions, procedures were gradually formulated, as the *skeletal outline* below demonstrates. The methods yielded, and continue to yield, successful results in every age group, from the three and a half right through the adult.

The two main spheres of work: IDENTIFICATION: BECOMING YOUR THEME AND EXTERNALIZATION: BECOMING YOUR THEME IN ACTION.

I:IDENTIFICATION: BECOMING YOUR THEME

A:PREPARATION

1. Re-orientation to Dance and to improvisation.

2. Building of concentration.

3. Practical work in disassociation of ideas concerning the human body (e.g. the re-education of the feet from their normal function of weight bearing and locomotion, to dance role of feet as an aorta of rhythm-emotion).

B. STIMULUS

1. Particularization, to pass beyond stale habit concept (e.g. animals are always a walk on all fours, until movement imagery is stirred by observation of specific characteristics, emotional state, etc.).

2. Limitation of theme (e.g. running through an obstacle, the movement reflecting the substance of the obstacle).

3. Finding the essence of an image for translation into movement.

4. Inter-transference of qualities between human body and the image.

5. Retention of the image by recall and association of ideas.

6. Build-up of atmosphere and role of accompaniment.

C. SOURCES OF IMAGERY

1. Structural images (e.g. extension of spinal span).

2. Spatial differentiation (e.g. animal in cage, in house, in field).

3. Time elements (e.g. retard or suddenness of weariness).

4. Realistic base: Rhythmic word action; Musical qualities (tremolo in action); Representational (the directness of rain): Stimulation by simulation (feeling dizzy); Similarity and Contrast; Pantomimic enactment; Emotion-action (the trembling, the stamping of foot in anger, etc.)

5. Action quotations from literature.

6. Associative ideas that intensify original stimulus (e.g. the adjective "light" like -- six year olds answer: pin, feather, paper, water, piece of thread).

7. Accessories (materials, objects, lights, pictures).

8. Authentic and derivative stimuli from folk and ethnic arts.

9. Accompaniment: silence, music, percussion, word patter.

NOTE: Sources of stimuli and imagery are only as effective as the teacher's method employed in their use.

D. CONTENT

1. The abstract, the specific, story themes, music interpretation, ethnic content, isolated elements of time, space and body movement as thematic content, social content, and the relative values of these.

2. Subject matter in relation to background, personality and age.

3. Length of improvisation and value of repetition.

4. Language: discussion guided by teacher: free verbalization.

II.EXTERNALIZATION: BECOMING YOUR THEME IN ACTION (e.g. our theme was feeling sleepy. First reaction of the children was to lie down still. We had to find the movements that expressed the feeling of wanting to lie down still).

A. ATTAINMENT OF SPONTANEITY

1. Fear, Convention, etc.

2. Unfamiliarity with the scope of instrument and medium.

B. POWER OF THE IMAGE AS A SOURCE OF ACTION STIMULUS

C. RELATION BETWEEN IMPROVISATION AND TECHNIQUE

1. Relation to skill and to set technical vocabulary and forms.

2. Relation to individual style; the questions of originality and effort.

OTHER THEORETICAL QUESTIONS:

Transference of freedom obtained to unguided creativity and performance before people; Relation to choreography; Inadequacies of improvisation for the contemporary student; Improvisation in its relation to creative release, and to therapy; Role of the teacher: kind and amount of beneficent control.

Let us take Point II B for illustration:

THE ANIMATED CLOTH

The highly developed imagination is, I believe, enormously related to the retention of mental images from life. This relation indicates the importance of developing retention of realistic images, and preceding that, clarification of the image. For example:

The children, a six to eight year group, were disorganized, rambunctious, inattentive. I said, "You are all so wild, would you like to do a wild dance?" "Yes", they shouted; but when the accompaniment commenced, they receded to the wall or sat down, only one or two making a stab at the improvisation. Faced with expression in terms of Dance, they felt utterly inadequate. My purpose was not to have a group made quiet through failure. I took a piece of cloth and asked them to watch *it* do a wild dance. To the same accompaniment, I manipulated the cloth with my hand, spasmodically into all directions. Some of them began to dance. No longer wild, nor inattentive; no longer disorganized, but concentrated, they were doing dances of wildness, moving in relation to an accompaniment, and using spatial levels and directions to express their theme. But two of them, one the shyest, the other the wildest, before the improvisation, were still plastered to the wall. I suggested each manipulate the little piece of cloth. The others noticed and all wanted it. We took enough pieces out of the Studio Chest, which contains varieties of real objects for stimulus from gentle bells to Oaxacan stone images. Each child manipulated a piece, and at just the right moment, as I had told them I would, I said, "let's drop the cloth and BE it". They did fine dances, and we could have proceeded to dances of wildness closer to human motivations.
The results so satisfied the children, we were able to go on to technical work, and to end our lesson in controlled, legato movement.

This particular experience illustrated several factors:

1. The disparity between emotion and the ability to express emotion in art.

2. The workability of a pedagogy of improvisation.

3. The close relation between the child's peace of mind, obtainable through creative release, and her ability to concentrate on technical problems.

4. The use of the moment as a springboard for constructive work. If your teaching is dynamic, new stimuli and methods are continually called forth by the material at hand.

THE SELF RELEASED

My objective had been to help students tap the essence of Dance. There were many unexpected by-products, which, in turn, broadened the pedagogy. I came to know the devices a child uses to reflect her inner feelings. For instance, by pretending, she expresses herself without calling forth ridicule, contempt or censure, from herself or the world. Not infrequently, she murders by proxy, and thus remains guilt free. An eight year old speaks: "In my dance, I had a dream. I was a prince and then someone came and told me my mother was dead--I was sad, but then I was happy again"--followed by (conscience speaking), -- "I don't know why". This child was able to dance out this death wish because it wasn't she, but she-the-prince-in-a-dream dance.

If a child does have a pent-up desire to dance out something, she will know how to utilize any suggested theme as a springboard. The same child so used the theme "Chinese Kites": "I was getting dead in the air, began to come down and tried to get back up. I tried and I tried and I tried, but in the end I came down and sank on the ground". This dance might aptly have been titled "Frustration" rather than "Chinese Kite"; a dance so emotionally true in its movement images, it would have been a rare treat on a concert program.

The children frequently used a suggested theme as a base for associative content. A girl of ten and a half, given the theme of "Hurricane", did a tortuous dance: "First I was the sleet, then I was a woman afraid of the sleet, then I was the sleet, then I was the woman in a hospital looking out of the window at the sleet, and it hit her and killed her".

Often a child will assume a role to attain the unattainable. A little girl of seven and a half sets a small stool in back center of the Studio. She hides behind it, slowly rises into view, and with original slow legato turns, describes a perfect circumference around the room; finishing in her first position, she disappears, sinking slowly behind the little stool. Pointing to it, she says, "This is a mountain. I am the Sun, rising and setting". Her dance is a dance of authority. Only its prelude and its epilogue, hiding behind "the mountain" expresses her littleness and timidity.

THE PLANT UPROOTED

Observing the children, it became clear that, once freed, certain themes recurred, related to age level. Two striking examples of adolescent personality found expression thus: One girl, on her knees, did a lovely Lotus Flower dance to Hindu music, while her explanation of it, (and of her stage in life) was: "I can't get away from my feet." Another, eleven and a half, used the theme of Sea Studies to mean this: "I was a plant -- a big wave came, knocked part of the plant off, so it was free. Another bigger wave, -- and the whole plant was uprooted and freed so it could dance anywhere in the water".

One of the most surprising discoveries of all was that rhythmic instability and technical limitations disappeared when the children engaged in improvisations. The inference that technical difficulties so often included factors of psychological conditioning, opened up new pedagogic vistas. The transformation of inadequacy into skill during the process of creative absorption, seems to indicate that *the instrument of dance, the body, is often a knotted skein, with impediments to technique and expressiveness entwined.*

The verbalizations quoted in this article were given of their own volition at the conclusion of the children's improvisations. Most often they dance without "telling their meaning", and when they did, I never questioned their content. GUIDANCE WITHOUT INTERFERENCE is the most important principle to follow. By relentlessly pursuing your objective, the "ordinary" student comes through, and, as of a sudden, her dancing takes on quality. *We know too little about the forces that nourish creativity to make snap judgments of a student's potentiality.*

The work described develops eventually a *self*-disciplined form of Dance, rich with the seed of creative renewal.

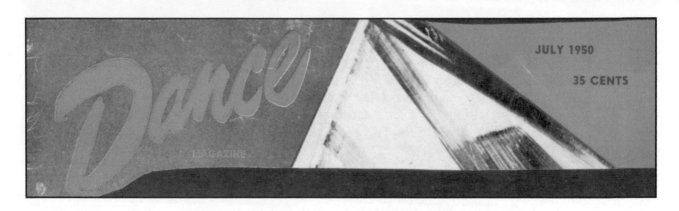

JULY 1950

35 CENTS

Butterflies and BOMBS!
the children dance life as THEY see it
article IX in the series

the CHILD'S WORLD: its relation to dance pedagogy

by Blanche Evan

In the Spring of 1949, at the conclusion of a lyrical lesson, a seven to ten year old class spontaneously made up the following for their favorite music, Tchaikovsky's *Waltz of the Flowers*: "We are beautiful wild flowers in the field, the wind comes and blows them almost to pieces. To the King of the flowers, the Wind says: 'I will stop blowing them only if you give me your fairest flower. If not, I will take you, the King and lock you up in my Wind castle.' The King figures out that, since he doesn't want to lose any of his flowers, nor be locked up in a castle, *he will make a fake flower, and put a bomb in it, give it to the wind, so when the wind takes it to the castle, it will blow up the whole thing, wind, castle, and all.* He does this!"

The American child of this generation is a War Child--a different kind of War Child from the hordes that overflow the abandoned debris shelters of Europe--but a war child nevertheless, who thinks in terms of atom bombs as well as fairy tales. In the last war, the children who attended dance class on Saturday, engaged in siren air raid drills in the public schools during the week, and wore their identification tags under their pretty practise costumes. Many sheltered relatives that had fled fascist persecution. Many felt abandoned by fathers and brothers called to service; and some came from homes where the war was discussed consciously to build hatred for fascism, personified by Hitler, Mussolini, and Hirohito.

It was a common sight to see kids on the street in New York engaging in pseudo-war--I have seen a child playing alone, taking both sides, the killer and the killed.

In this atmosphere of extremest tension, there were theatre groups for children that became more pink-stained than ever, to divert the child from the horrors of the world,--as if they could! Such an attitude greatly minimizes the impact on the child of the adult world, laid bare to the child by every means of communication open to the adult.

The children need help in relating to the *real* world, they need creative channels in which to relieve the burden that our distraught adult world has placed upon their little shoulders; and they, as well as the adult, need a connecting link between the adult's tensions and their own.

With all this in mind, between the years of 1941 and 1945, I led the children to the creation of many dances indirectly and directly related to the war. Through Dance, they found constructive outlet for their pent-up feeling, and *explored all the facets of tenderness and brutality the material held for them.* Because we faced reality though the children's senses, their dances, emerging in semi-improvisational, semi-compositional form, were as true to the nature of children in style and contour, as their more usual dances of simple exuberance.

GESTAPO

Phyllis, age 11, contributed an original script, *Gestapo*:

"An English flier grounded in Germany is rescued by an anti-fascist German woman. The Gestapo, who finds them, throws them into a concentration camp, and tries in vain to get information from the German woman, even torturing the flier before her eyes. The dance ends with the woman defiantly refusing to be intimidated. Moral: not even torture can compel assistance to the Nazis."

We used an old piece of wooden partition for the "concentration camp", and percussion for accompaniment. In this particular dance, the children never wanted to change roles with each other, because each of them found such tremendous satisfaction for *personal* needs, in the parts they originally chose.

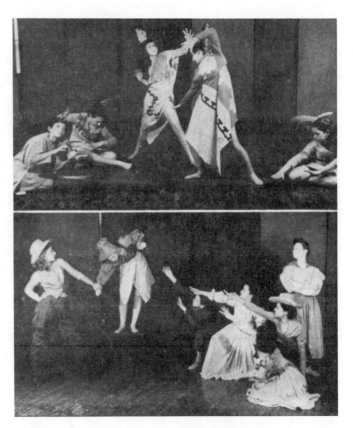

History became alive — as adolescence found release. (Two sequences from ON FREEDOM ROAD).

PEARL HARBOR

Pearl Harbor, (1943), created by Monita, and Rena Gluck, both nine years, was a duet in three parts: *Planting Rice, The Bombs Fall,* and--*You Will Pay for This*--as Monita listens to the silenced heart beat of her co-worker. The trio Gestapo was heroic, the duet *Pearl Harbor* utterly poignant.

One of the ballets employed fantasy to sharpen the children's awareness of the world in which they lived: "The Dragon Meets the People" (1941), centered around the symbolic figure of the three headed monster of fascism.

TOWER OF VICTORY

Since adolescent dances almost always concern themselves with love, in *Tower of Victory*, (1944), we used a love theme as the base:

"A European peasant boy and girl are being feted at their wedding ceremony, when the Nazis raid their town. The ballet develops along the lines of the cruel domination of the invaders, and the determination of the villagers, whose shrewdness and courage effect their liberation. There follows the intense communal reconstruction of their town, the search for the lost ones, the beautiful reunion of the lovers, with the wedding celebration completed at the end."

The plot gave plenty of scope to the creators for their innermost, and seemingly contradictory emotional needs. For instance, some of the girls asked for several parts, switching from the cruel Nazis to the courageous villagers. The children suggested and developed characters and scenes: the very restrained comic drunk episode of two Nazi guardsmen; and the woman who turns spy out of personal revenge for the loss of her husband in battle. The dance, *Return to Life*, succeeding the Battle, was an exquisite sensitive dance, the search for each other, and the slow awareness of sun and the imperishable effort to live. I shall never forget Iris (the storm trooper of two years previous), as she wandered around, slowly touching walls, and lovingly lifting imagined objects from the earth, as she danced the character she created--a woman turned gently mad with grief. There were also Cecile's charming *A Child Dances*, and Rena's intense study, *Strength*. And one of the most touching dances I have ever seen, by the eight year olds, *The Children Will Never Forget*. I contributed simple choreographic forms to bind the whole together, as in *Building the Tower* that marked the victory of the villagers. In the main, the children's movements were their own, and they danced as personality, age, and understanding demanded. We bought no costumes, and we performed the ballet at an informal afternoon for the parents. It had eleven dances, and ran for forty consecutive minutes.

ON FREEDOM ROAD

On Freedom Road, (1945), was a sequence of dances by a group of twelve and thirteen year olds. It was based on three episodes in American history: the closing in of the American Indian, emancipation of the Negro slave, and allies of world war II. When these adolescent girls danced history, they were also dancing personal feelings of bondage and freedom. Their conflicts between their need to be free, and their lingering dependence on the parent, found, unbeknown to their conscious selves, satisfying outlet in the dances of the Auction Sale of Slaves, and the Emancipation Dance to Lincoln's Proclamation. On the other hand, their identification deepened their understanding of the social content of this ballet. We used source material like Howard Fast's pro-American-Indian book, and excerpts from Lincoln's inspired speeches. We used an authentic American Indian music, recorded on location, and bought some basic material at eight cents a yard, which Marion, one of the group, painted in striking Indian designs. We danced to Negro Spirituals, and to the indigenous folk music of our allies: of the Soviet Union and of England. The three periods of history were bound thematically by the struggle for freedom.

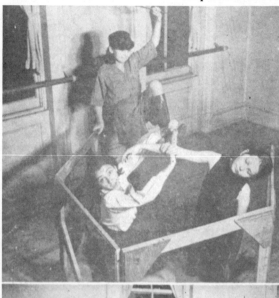

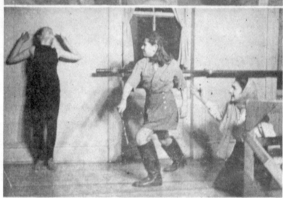

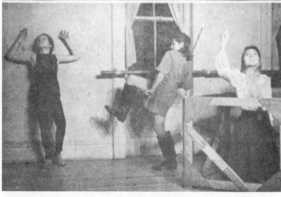

In these dances related to WAR, the children chose their won parts. Through identification with social content, they found tremendous outlet for their own personality needs. In GESTAPO, highly imaginative Iris (age 10), chose the part of the brutal Nazi storm trooper. Neatrice (age 9) shy and sensitive, developed the role of the tortured captive, while Phyllis (age 11) who originated the plot, took the part of the valiant woman.

COAL

One of the finest realistic ballets the children ever danced was the *Story of Coal*: "deep under the ground, where the miners work in pits..." The booklet we used as source material contained what to us was surprising information, and demonstrated again, how close to the child's world, material of social content can be: For instance, "...a canary is part of the equipment of every mine. When there is danger, the little bird is overcome by the gas long before the men even become aware of it--and so the warning is given." Who would ever dream of canaries in coal mines?

Fairy tales? They are wonderful--but let the child dance them after she has a footing in reality--not before, when the footing may be so insecure that she will find she has slipped from the turret of her fancies only to crash to the hard pavements of our modern world. The child's world of fantasy today includes bombs as well as butterflies. The tensions that result can find release in creativity that does not turn from, but rather faces this fact. This does not lessen the child's joy,--rather clears the blocks for joy to come through.

Even the most stark material of the adult world today is common knowledge among children and this material contains wide scope for identification. The use of this material in the creative dance class, where the child can involve her body in the turbulent rhythms of *our* times, helps to form a positive bond between the child's and the adult's world. Also--and this is no mean advantage--it gives the teacher the opportunity to exert positive influence interpreting what otherwise may well remain darkness and fear--or, even worse, what may become to the child a twentieth century acceptance of destructiveness.

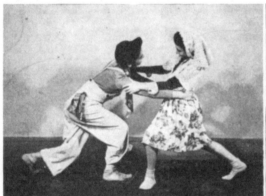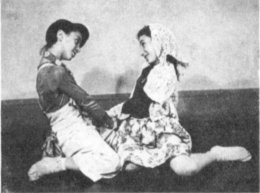

Adolescents always dance of love. Simple forms were used to bind the whole together, as in "building the tower". (Four scenes from the TOWER OF VICTORY.)

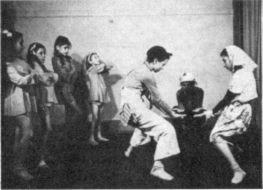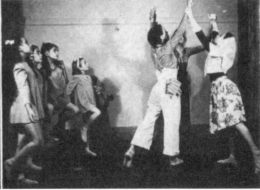

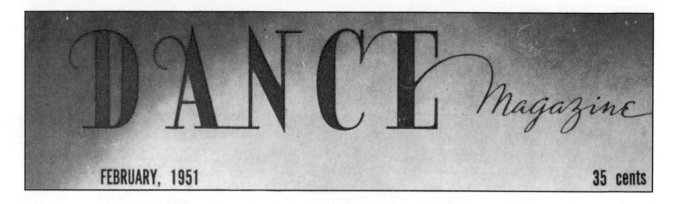

FEBRUARY, 1951   35 cents

THE SOURCE conclusion of the series:
THE CHILD'S WORLD
its relation to
dance pedagogy
by Blanche Evan

Editor's Note

This is the last article in this particular series in which Blanche Evan has been presenting what she considers fundamental issues in teaching creative dance to children. The following is a list of the nine preceding installments:

January 1949: *Defining the Child's World*, February 1949: *The Child's Need*, March 1949: *The Link Between*, May 1949: *Re-Orientation and Posture*, July 1949: *Heart Beat*, November 1949: *Rhythm of Sharing*, January 1950: *Who Is Everybody*, March 1950: *I Am The Sun*, July 1950: *Butterflies — and Bombs*.

Re-Education

The inborn urge to express emotion in rhythmic body movement makes dance world over a natural activity. Our own culture neglects and tends to destroy this natal potential for dance. The teacher's task is to restore it and to *re-educate* the body to a state wherein movement response functions. In this process of *re-education*, the teacher can extend the natural endowments into an experience of art in terms of the child's own environment.

Newell: "True child's play is a sacred mystery at which their elders can only obtain glances by stealth through the crevice of the curtain ...."

To restore and to build, we must have knowledge of the normal child's first orientations to movement. Where are we to seek this knowledge? The psychologists and pediatricians are as yet unfamiliar with the specifics of the art of dance, while the dance teachers are not humble enough before the child.

NO ADULT DANCER CAN POSSIBLY KNOW THE NATURAL PROPENSITIES OF DANCE IN CHILDREN EXCEPT BY OBSERVING CHILDREN THEMSELVES UNDER CONDITIONS OF RELATIVE FREEDOM AND IN AN ATMOSPHERE AS RELAXED AS POSSIBLE.

Our work requires observing them in every stage of growth: in their cribs, in their free play on the streets, on the beaches, at times when they think they are unobserved; and in the dance class itself as they react to the work they are taught, and as they contribute to the class.

Your class then becomes your laboratory. What you discover is more valid for use than other contributory sources. Study of movement in animals, in the whole realm of nature, study of psychology, of anatomy, and of indigenous dance are certainly worthwhile, but *the most productive source for materials and methods is the child herself.*

To Discover, to Restore, to Build

With the youngest group of three to six years, we have the opportunity to explore the true potentialities of creative dance in conditions of our own culture. This gives us a standard by which to determine the environmental deviations and developments manifested as the child grows older.

In the realm of physical technique, I have observed the following:

1. *The younger the child, the more immediate is her response to rhythm.* (See Articles 5 & 6)

2. *The young child without adult direction explores body movement for heightening movement prowess.*

Recently I watched a child of nineteen months accidentally roll from a little stool into a somersault. He then repeated the process half a dozen times, with obvious delight, but from the second time on, accident became intention. He had sat himself at the edge of the stool *in order to* achieve the somersault.

3. *The young child, given a lead, naturally widens movement experience with a startling, intuitive logic.* Sitting on the floor, the 4-year olds were being directed to "making spaces" between toes, then fingers. When they stood up, without any word from the teacher, they began to widen the foot base with "look at my big spaces, look at me make a big space", as they spread into a very wide 2nd. How much more significance this held for them than if the teacher had said: "Now children, put your feet apart".

In tune with children, a good approach to their technical development, includes the leeway for teacher and child to develop technical movement, *within the class hour*, in a successive manner, similar to free association in thought.

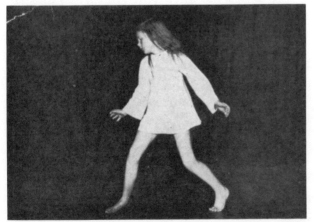
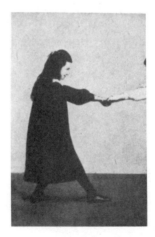

Student at the Blanche Evan school of Creative Dance — taken in action by Fred Fehl, 1950.

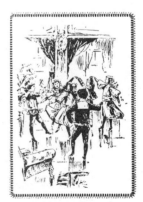

Children dancing in 1898.

4. *In locomotion the growing child seeks the experience of extending movement into space at first horizontally, then vertically.* The dance studio floor therefore assumes a role of tremendous importance as a physical-emotional base.

The floor level plays a big role in the struggle of the child in growing up. It should be utilized not only as a place for "stretches", but also as ground for reexploring navigational possibilities. It is also a place to return to from the standing level with its strains of balance, returning in movement to the floor level endeared to the child as the first home in foreign space away from her mother's arm.

5. *The child evolves in movement* from lying supine to crawling, rolling, climbing, standing, walking-running, jumping, galloping, skipping. Skipping comes at least two years after galloping. Leaping, demanding height <u>with</u> breadth *with* transference of weight in the air, demands specific dance skill. Even for the nine and ten year olds, it should follow a long succession of mastery of simpler forms of locomotion.

6. *The child in the process of becoming upright loses specific flexibilities and strengths* not necessarily for functional reasons, but because in our society she is forced to restrict them. For instance, a young child has extensive use of the muscles in the groin and upper thigh which she manifests by sitting comfortably with thighs turned either in or out. The adults in Oriental and equatorial cultures retain this by the positions they assume in the home and in their work. Our children lose it, and because of the stress in our society and in dance technique of the straight stance, they develop stiff knees and inadequate flexion in the groin and ankle.

The teacher needs to devise technical forms to waylay this petrification of movement.

7. *Children's feet in even the youngest groups show the structuring* effects of the shoe and the unresilient cement and wood grounds.

The child needs counter-active exercise in the separate joints of the feet.

According to Dr. W. M. Phelps' theory ("Diagnosis for Treatment of Postural Defects") foot weakness in children are transferred more directly than any other deficiencies to the postural weakness of the adult.

8. *The very young child in contrast to the adult, naturally uses the body as a mobile structure,* wherein units of the body *respond* to other units functionally, for the preservation of balance. A child first does a back bend sitting on her knees, head way back, the spine arched, buttocks extended to the back. Standing, she eliminates the head thrust. This young child might be able to do a complete back bend to the floor with hips forward, but only with terrific strain, and possibly injury, since the movement would be in opposition to the spinal mobility which naturally absorbs strains at that age. A full back bend would force it into a position of equilibrium for which the child is physically and psychologically unprepared.

Technique such as complete back bends should not be taught until the child's spine functions with more solidity, although it is constructive to teach simple exercises for the strengthening of the spinal muscles.

A great deal of the movement given the child should permit rather than destroy the reflex-like response of the joints, so sorely lacking in adults. This automatically eliminates most of the adult techniques of rigid controls.

9. *The very young child uses torsal movement at first from a position of relatively easy balance.* We should not expect too much from the child in torsal movements in conjunction with difficult

forms of locomotion, when logically, most of her concentration would be on the problems of balance and weight transference.

Furthermore, locomotion, to the child, has a *special purpose* relating to going somewhere, to pursuit, to exuberance, to sports; which brings us to the discussion of the relationship between the play forms of children and their dancing.

PART II

The "Sacred Mystery"

It took me many years to understand why our children considered a dance circle as something to break into, to break away from, or to destroy, until I found that most *athletic games in circle form* possess as their dominating characteristic the *dissolution* of the circle. Of the thirty-five circle games I investigated, only one -- of Africa -- stresses the cohesiveness of the circle.

In cultures where the community dance is part of life, the child grows up using games to express the excitements of chance and competition, balancing this outlet with communal dance controlled by rhythm and content and the social life. Our children, lacking communal dance, can credit to their experience only the movement and philosophy of games. This is their equipment when they commence their study of dance.

If we seek the source of movement within the child, the meaning of movement in the world of play merits thorough investigation. To understand the games they love, those that are universal, those that are specific to our environment, -- to understand this enables us directly to change the child's limited orientation to movement enlarging it to the realm of dance. It also gives the dance teacher insight into those *secrets of movement behavior* so precious to children (and sometimes so disturbing to the teacher.)

Certain forms of play are found in all cultures including our own, among which are the games based on pure skill in body movement, with little or no equipment, like the many varieties of hopping, running and jumping. The spatial patterns enlisted by children in these games are varied and interesting: patterns of snakes, spirals, loops, boxes and lines. The large patterns are similar in outline to those of folk dance and may have similar origin. In any case, children love them. Technique employing spatial formations of seemingly intrinsic interest might offer a means to the teacher of adding meaning to "the step", of increasing the child's handling of space, and of breaking the monotonous use of the diagonal in class work.

One of our most direct transitions to "abstract" co-ordination lies in the springboard use of movement derived from the child's world of play with equipment: the dipping movement of ice skating, the controlled symmetry of the see-saw, the scooping crescendo of the swing, the repetitive rotations of the jumping rope, the top and the merry-go-round. Please note the words "springboard", "derived from", etc. Nothing is so puerile as naturalistic imitations by the human body of objects and animals and movement phenomenon.

Indeed, did you ever *see* the wind?

In a psychological sense, do we not have something important to learn from the doggerels of humor and comment which the child, in a most detached manner, composes *to accompany movements requiring real skill*--as in the O'Leary ball game with it's *twenty-two* movement sequences; and from their love for the *rhythm of a sound* where common sense is *indicated*, despite, or because of, (can we judge?) the "non-sensical".

"I know a man named Michael Finnegan
He wears whiskers on his chinnnegan.
Along came a wind and blew them in again;
Poor old Michael Finnegan, begin again."

Transition

"Beginnings offer the surest footholds... what features have changed? Which are preserved? Which are lost? What are the new impulses?" (Gideon).

In the technique of creative dance for children, the teacher has to carry the child through many transitional stages of discovery and growth; and from the restored natural propensity of movement to the realm skill specific to the art of Dance.

If we can develop a technique that recaptures for the growing child the germ of satisfaction she manifested in beating time to music in infancy; the kind of thrill she knew when she increased her range of movement from level to level; and the joy she felt at sharing movement in her first acts of social play, we can be sure we are tapping the child's inborn equipment for dance technique.

Fused with this primary orientation to Dance, each age group has a typical movement response which a searching teacher comes to recognize and which should be utilized as a source for shaping the child's technique. Three years old may love to roll on the floor whereas eleven year olds want to work on posture. Six to eight year olds can never find music fast enough in a kind of perpetual motion frenzy, whereas the adolescent responds better to technical movement with an inherent climactic pattern.

If we accept the premise that the source *is* the child, the basis of training from the age of three to nine is the same regardless of professional intent. The undisputed presence of great gift, -- a phenomenon not too frequent, -- would not change the basis for training, although it would certainly influence its intensity and rate of progress. This series has limited itself to the Dance as an activity complete in its own realm for the dancing child of non-professional purpose. Though few may engage in Dance professionally, dancing continues for them in one form or another as an enduring part of their lives.

In closing the series, I should like to tell my readers that I have felt an enormous responsibility in presenting this material that grew out of my own observations and personal experience. I want to thank them, the teachers, parents, and dancers, whose response and enthusiasm lends warm encouragement to this work of endless challenge. Teaching children creative dance is as deep and far reaching as children themselves.

The children of my own School of Creative Dance have been the main material for my experiments and the main source of my inspiration. I should like to end the series in the words of one of them, a nine-year old, who, without premeditation, wrote the following in class:

What dancing means to me:

"Dancing to me, is not only one of my weekly practices, but is also a time for using my imagination. Dancing helps me to build up muscles. It is a time to do what I want up to a certain point. It is a time to learn about the world dancers and their history. Dancing allows me to describe my thoughts as well as I can. I think that it really helps me understand." ...Betsy

Something about the author of

THE CHILD'S WORLD

Blanche Evan has to her credit a total of over twenty articles published on dance by Dance Magazine, Dance Observer, American Dancer, Parents Magazine, Theatre Arts Monthly, etc. Her first article appeared in Theatre Arts in 1935; caused a storm in the modern dance world, due to her candour in relating personal experiences in studying with two of the "great" modern schools of the day.

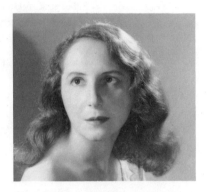

The author, Miss Blanche Evan.

Miss Evan made her professional debut at the age of 7 1/2 at the old Century Theatre in New York City, attired as a lettuce leaf. At the age of nine decided to devote the rest of her life to dance. She did. Left ballet school at the ripe age of fourteen in search of a more creative form. Found Bird Larson; studied with her two years. The latter's death left Miss E. forlorn and with out direction. From this point, she followed her own bent, searching for a technique and expression not taught in other schools of that day.

Commenced college after Miss Larson's death; spent lunch hours on roof, dancing for student friends. Decided college was not for her when she nearly failed gym course because of her resistance to a dance called "Sleigh Bells", which she refused to learn.

Gave many solo performances, lectures and demonstrations between 1932 and 1947, when illness cut short all professional appearances.

Opened her own school in 1934 with two children and ten adults as students. Last year, she had an enrollment of 150 children and 24 adults.

Was very active in dance guilds and associations, and in efforts to educate the public to dance. Invented free course for men in active dance appreciation. One of the first applicants to enroll was a boy named MICHAEL KIDD, who studied with her for two years. His daughter, Kristine, 3 1/2 years old, is now her student. Another young dancer who has achieved some small celebrity locally, RENA GLUCK, spent seven years in Miss Evan's class.

She has travelled extensively, and seen native dance in the Balearic Isles of Spain. in the U.S.S.R., the voladores in Papantla, Mexico, the reels and Highland Fling in the Scottish colony of Cape Breton and the rumba in Cuba's interior.

DANCE OBSERVER

VOLUME TWENTY-SIX, NUMBER NINE   NOVEMBER, 1959

THERAPEUTIC ASPECTS OF CREATIVE DANCE
Brief comments on a Weighty Subject
by Blanche Evan

THE STUDENT This article refers to "the student" rather than "the patient" because it deals with Creative Dance as Therapy *in the dance studio* in the non-psychotic.

Creative Dance as a people's activity has therapeutic values for the healthy, the "normally disturbed," the neurotic, the psychotic and the disabled. Although all five share the values of physical reconditioning and "psycho-kinaesthetic" reward, the *responses* of the five categories to the same material are distinctly different. An effective teacher in this work relates pedagogic substance to the students' "psycho-physical" condition.

Demarcation is necessary in the range of the physical, psychological, and kinaesthetic even though the very reason for "C D" as Therapy is their ultimate unification . For example, a healthy person accepts pelvic movement in the usual course of a lesson, whereas the neurotic and psychotic often react so subjectively that the consequent rendition is distorted with sexual frustration or supercharged with abandonment. Another example; a neurotic obese student will do the same stretch as a normal weight person but the physical state of obesity will have caused the student to become overly shy and very low in "body self-esteem." To her the accomplishment of the stretch will mean an extension of personal worth whereas the normal weight person at best will complain that her hamstrings hurt . Again: an improvisation to sad music seemed the right choice for one class, but one of the students referred by a therapist went home and cried the whole night. The innocuous music had touched off the physical outlet -- of tears.

STUDENT CATEGORIES: I. *Normally healthy student*: A study of expression *through one's own body, not* passively watching someone else dance on the concert stage, acts as catharsis and can add up to preventive therapy. A person who lets out along the way has more of a chance of being on even keel than one who, "society-bound," holds in at the price of "cumulative frustration." 2. The loneliness typical of today may find a modicum of comfort in expressive movement in the C D class. 3. Many other therapeutic gains too numerous to mention here.

II. *"Normally disturbed"* is my own term (as are the other designations in quotes) to describe the person of our time who rejects the blatant characteristics of contemporary society, who is harassed by the noise, the megalomania, the success story UNATTAINABLE for most, who is aghast at the violence, the junior delinquency and the adult atom bomb, who as a result is often depressed, discouraged, confused. The prevalent person of our time profits therapeutically in C D especially when the teacher utilizes CONTENT that makes contact with the hurt areas. I separate these "social neuroses" from personality problems of the individual neurotic student.

Note: The American modern dance has demonstrated in practice two marked American Standards: the one of mass conformity, the other of individualism stemming from the each-one-for-himself ideology of democracy. In dealing with the "normally disturbed" in C D we are in part dealing with the consequences of this schizoid social attitude to the body of the individual ego.

III. <u>The Neurotic Student.</u> I arbitrarily confine this category to the adult who has or is undergoing psychotherapy and who has either sought out the C D studio on her own or who has been recommended by her therapist to the activity as an adjunctive therapy. Occasional contact exist between therapist and dance teacher. As a rule the student carries back to her therapy session relevant material about herself that had found its way to the surface in her dance hour. Of

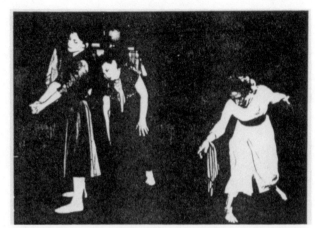

Teachers under Miss Evan's supervision in an improvisation. The theme assigned is "Restless".

course there are many dance students who are neurotic but who have not undergone psychotherapy. There is a *distinct difference* in the dance work of the neurotic who has *not*, or who *has been* or *is* in the process of psychotherapy. The latter is apt to employ far greater resistance and to repeat some of the transference mechanisms of psychotherapy to the dance teacher. Because she lives on inner melodrama and evasion, she is subject to greater inhibition in true improvisation. She manifests sensitivity of a very subjective nature and has surprisingly keen insight into the Dance objectives. One student wrote; <u>Movement for me began like a sort of stuttering of the body...and became an awareness of earthly locomotion...to stand and walk...without disturbance.</u>" The neurotic adult frequently indulges in *unselfconscious* verbalization in the dance class: "I feel like killing someone tonight but it won't be you" one student whispered to my assistant who had been assigned to be her partner. The same young woman another night said, "It takes an awful lot to give me the feeling that life may be a nice, happy, joyful thing after all ...and essentially I...feel that way after a class."

IV. *Dance for the psychotic patient* in the hospital setup is not included in this article.

V. C D *for the Disabled* 1. The normal disability: for example, one student referred to me had broken both ankles in WAC service during the war and had developed a block to walking, although both ankles had regained almost complete mobility. 2. The mentally retarded, the blind, deaf, cerebral palsy. A few individual teachers, like Ruth Benov, who devotes some of her teaching time to the retarded, are doing fine experimental work on their own. The C D teacher can increase the range of body movement of many disabled by way of muscular renewal and expressive vitality *that no other activity* affords them. The teacher should discover not only what compensatory mechanisms the disabled have developed UNKNOWN to the normal person.

THE TEACHER: *Negative.* Creative Dance as Therapy, as a new field, is attracting many teachers, college dance majors, and even teen age dancers, some of whom are surely sincere. Nevertheless, I am reminded of how teachers jumped on the band wagon of C D for children about ten years ago exploiting the fruits of the few who had done the pioneer dredging out of dedication to art and to educational progress. Many newcomers reaped the benefits in money and today are teaching one or another form of mangled C D in popularized versions that are neither creative nor dance. The dance teacher who is an opportunist in the field of dance therapy should be warned that it is criminal to deal with therapy in any form without acquiring background.

2. The modern dance teacher who treats a class of students as so many automatons to acquire perfection in stylistic movement stemming from the academic modern dance schools, has no place in the use of movement as therapy. 3. The teacher who regards the whole process of "self-expression" in Dance as a somewhat embarrassing phenomenon also should remove herself from the scene of the therapist's field.

POSITIVE: Therapy means help. If a dance teacher really wants to employ her art to benefit the student in terms of the living problem before her, the following are what I believe to be basic musts for the teacher:

1. She must reorient herself to the art of Dance as a therapeutic tool in every aspect--and yet *she must continue to revere her art and to cherish it as her mainspring of inspiration.*

2. She must seek the bodily dance experience *herself* of that CONTENT that relates to Dance as therapy. No self-respecting analyst gives analysis without having undergone analysis himself. An analogy can be drawn to the dance teacher who should experience Dance as therapy as a new entity before giving it out or drawing it out of others.

3. She must develop a new awareness of "emotional-physical tonus" as a factor to be dealt with in the student.

4. She must develop a new orientation to thematic material, to its tremendous potential in therapeutic work and to its manipulation in improvisation. The selection and malleable use of content by teachers is the weakest sphere of pedagogy in C D today.

5. She must read or go to school to get a background of psychotherapy.

THE THERAPIST The therapeutic, educational and medical professions are slowly becoming dance conscious. These include psychotherapists, both psychiatrists and psychologists, practitioners in education, social work, child guidance workers, physicians including orthopedists, and surgeons. A few in each field realize that Creative Dance, or at the least body movement, has salutary factors for their patients and they do make private referrals.

A Psychiatric Center in Kansas set a precedent this autumn in giving a grant to one of its nurses to study Dance Therapy with the writer. Now Creative Dance is scheduled 3 hours daily for their patients and another hour for the nurses.

Here and there one does find an institutional budget for dance for the disabled and the psychotic. I know of no clinic for *neurotic* patients that has an allotment to further collaborative work between therapist and dance teacher or that pays a dance therapist on the staff. And most dance therapists work so purely by chance and without psychotherapeutic background that they cannot in all truth command a salary. I have even met some who seem to feel that because they are dealing with the sick they themselves do not have to have much dance proficiency in order to teach.

All this may sound discouraging for the honest dance therapist who is drawn to the work for itself and who needs to make a living by it. Actually the more *people* who dance C D in any of the five categories as I have classified them, are by a natural process spreading the "message" of the constructive contribution of Creative Dance to our society where orbit and jet and nuclear power, mechanical science--and the baseball bat have all but obliterated the power of the body to speak for itself.

How does "Dance therapy differ from movement therapy?

Following is an unpublished case of mine which by example clearly indicates that the decision of choice rests upon the needs of the client and how best these needs can be met by the media of movement or Dance or Both. This was a very successful case yet the client never danced in session.

THE PSYCHOPHYSICAL COMPONENTS ARE IN ANY CASE VITAL.

"FANNY"
by Blanche Evan

In 1960, one thousand reprints of my article "THERAPEUTIC ASPECTS OF CREATIVE DANCE" (Dance Observer - Nov. 1959) were circulated. One of the most interesting responses come from a staff psychologist in a rehabilitation center for children from broken homes in Brooklyn. "This sounds just right for my thirteen year old client. Could she have some sort of social dancing where she can mix with people her own age?"

My interview with the girl led me to believe that she could benefit by body movement and Dance in private sessions on a level completely different from social dancing. From the start I had the full cooperation of the counselor and the institution --and the client.

Fanny (so we shall call her) was physically ill: a polio-scoliosis case. Parents had been divorced. She was living with her mother and step-father both of whom had full time jobs. She had dropped out of school though she was a very bright girl. Certainly here was a web of physical-psychological-social problems, the weight of the world on the diseased back of a sensitive adolescent.

Of my own volition, through contact with the social worker at Fanny's scoliosis treatment clinic, I visited her medical doctor. Dr. G. verified my observations as to Fanny's limitations of gluteal musculature, her uncontrolled scapular range, and what the doctor termed her knock knees and flat feet. He gave me liberty to go ahead except, because of the spinal fusion, to avoid extreme spinal stretches and lateral movement. He was not too hopeful of the benefit of exercise in view of the enormous amount of impairment, but I "could try" and he would be interested in the results.

The results were achieved not through Dance but through functional exercise based on individual need coupled with my objective to help Fanny change her attitude from passive defeat to a realistic attitude to the impairment itself.

For example Fanny had told me of the repeated experience at night walking in a panic not able to straighten out her left leg. I suggested she move the "good" leg at such times and then the other. The panic was thereby lessened. Then she felt it straightened too much! We worked on the problem until she understood something about spasm, which might be helped through heat. Her mother cooperated with a heating pad and Dr. G. suggested soaking in hot tubs. What had seemed to Fanny like an evil spell now became a physical problem to be handled therapeutically.

Fanny had great difficulty climbing stairs. The effort was always accompanied by fatigue with pounding, throbbing headache. I worked out exercises that approximated stair climbing which she added to her home practice. As the muscles gained strength and the mechanism of weight transfer was understood by her, the physical strain was lessened, her awkwardness decreased -- and the headaches disappeared entirely! Climbing stairs will never be easy for her but she is now relieved of the throbbing tensions, some of the physical fatigue, and of the emotional strain of being conspicuously disabled in public.

At this point I shall submit to the reader some self-explanatory excerpts from my final report to Fanny's counselor:

FIRST LESSON	LAST LESSON
Psoas muscles utterly weak. "The physical therapist used to get angry and tell me I had no stomach muscles."	Now is able to execute one of the most difficult exercises dependent for execution almost solely on these muscles.
Knock knees	Now controlled through corrective exercise
Did not know how to move her toes	Now has developed a beautiful point
Could not balance standing on 2 feet No power to lift leg to the back	Now is able to balance for minutes poised on one leg with other leg lifted in high arabesque. Can now ride in subway in rush hour holding packages maintaining balance without leaning on anything and without fear
In order to sit down on floor, tremendous contortion and great fear of falling	Now descends to floor gracefully and inconspicuously. Fanny is greatly relieved as to her motor appearance on the beach this coming summer
Fear of falling while bending forward and while walking	Now replaced by positive confidence both in static position and in locomotion.
Inability to run and jump based on fear, lack of technique, and on constant overstress of weight on right leg due to impairment of left	Now runs many times around studio without pause; spontaneously hops without support. Conscious effort now NOT to spare left leg but to make it take weight and to work wherever possible, resulting in better equilibrium; and for facing up to the impairment rather than coddling it
"When I walk, my body seems to be in front and my legs behind me"	"My body is one now. It is unified".

X-rays were due coinciding in time with the end of our sessions. It was a great day when Dr. G. had Fanny walk before him without her brace. (He had allowed her to go without her brace during sessions with me). She walked beautifully, straight, and with an air of self-support. Dr G. said she may soon be able to dispense with her brace permanently.

Fanny has an uncanny kinaesthetic insight rarely found in our culture. This combined with her conscientious daily practice and intelligence were important factors in her remarkable progress.

In our last session, in discussing the whole question of equilibrium in stance, Fanny commented: "Yes, when one is unevenly balanced, or unbalanced, one feels so" --I was sure she was going to say `insecure' but she didn't; she said, "one feels so -- insignificant!"

I had helped Fanny to distinguish between what she thought her body could NOT do from the reality of what it COULD do. This process included reference to those body actions that were difficult for all bodies, normal as well as disabled. I had helped her to face up to the reality of her impairment as a factor of realistic behavior with a conscious utilization of her present body potential, to the full. She said: "I felt as if my body was wasting away...My legs were rotting away -- now I know I can lift a leg". In the middle of an exercise she would exclaim: "I did it, I did it, I did it!"

Although we had not had Dance lessons as such, on the last day she said, "I really look good when I walk. I don't even remember how clumsy I was. Today I had so much energy, I had to do something with it -- I danced it out. I never used to feel this way. I never wanted to move about at all."

SUMMARY CONCLUSIONS

It is very important to establish contact with the client's counselors, social workers, doctors, therapists, even when circumstances compel minimal exchange of ideas and information yielded.

The objective of increased health should deal with the reality of the 24 hour day that the client lives.

No work done therapeutically in the field of body movement or Dance can be separated from the psychological components. The Dance therapist should open the work to what I term EMPHASIS NEED: Clarify the objective, then work with the clay and let a shape come to life, rather than pour your clients' needs into a prepared mould with shape preordained.

Dance-body movement-therapy has an immeasurable contribution to make to health on diverse social, psycho-physical, educational levels. It has just barely begun to push its first stem through the hard encrustation of society's attitudes to the body itself.

June 1960.

dance

magazine

march, 1952

35 cents

the dancer of Pompeii
by blanche evan

Dancers of this generation made their first acquaintance with ancient Greek dance by way of the photos and drawings of the American Isadora Duncan dancing in Greek tunics. For those of us who never saw Duncan dance, it was not easy to understand the phenomenon of a twentieth century American finding roots in ancient Greece. As I travelled through the Greek ruins of Sicily this past summer, I felt I was able to make emotional contact with the qualities of unity and classical permanence sought by Duncan in ancient Greek art. Especially was this true as I fell spell bound before the perfect Doric temple of Segesta, standing intact through all these centuries in the solitude of the Sicilian hills.

Continuing through the magnificent museums of Naples, Pompeii, Florence and Rome, I came upon paintings, murals and statuary of ancient Greek and Renaissance dance that I had never seen reproduced. One of the most beautiful was the "Danzatrice of Tivoli" in the National Museum of Rome, a statue that, despite the demolished head and arms, embodies the roundness and expansive breadth characteristic of the best in "free" dance.

In extreme contrast were the six large archaic brown-green bronzes that stand on a long marble bench in the Naples Museum. They are the "Attrice e Danzatrice" of Herculaneum, the pupils of their eyes black on the white eye ball, staring through twenty five centuries of time. Their straight unyielding lines bear comparison with the three impressive panels of the "Danza Rituale" from the tombs of Ruva, paintings whose colors of yellow, white, black, red and blue, are not so fresh as the Pompeiian frescos, but nevertheless distinguishable and three dimensional in effect. The tiny black and white outline of this work, figure 530 in Maurice Emanuel's " Antique Greek Dance", truly depreciates the grandeur of these huge oblong originals that cover three sides of a spacious room.

I was struck by the numbers of dancing statues of satyrs, children and bacchantes holding percussion instruments in their hands: cymbals, flutes, drums, tambourines; and remembered again that Duncan seemed to have avoided the unadorned sounds of percussion both in her dances and in their accompaniment. The accompanying illustration is described in one catalogue as "Ganimede and Faun carrying the Bacchus boy on its shoulders".

The bronze "Fauno Danzante", now in Naples Museum, originally marking the entrance to the Casa Fauna in Pompeii, captures an ecstatic moment in dance.

Pompeii--the resurrected silent city that holds the traveller spell bound. When I saw the deposits of black lava on Mount Etna, and the houses of the neighboring villages built of the huge blocks of petrified fire, it was not difficult to imagine a whole city buried and simultaneously preserved under its solid flowing masses. As you walk on the huge stones of the Pompeiian streets, cleft by chariot wheels, you know indeed that you are walking into the past, your feet treading the very stones where Greek and Roman sandals trod two thousand years before you.

The House of Vitteii is one of the largest in Pompeii. The walls of one of the "cubicula", a small room adjoining the open court, are covered with frescoes, their colors still fresh: beautiful yellows, luminous greens and Pompeiian red. There are the exquisite "Amorini" in actions of "Work and Play" and the "Fauni Funamboli" that together might well be a children's ballet. Some of the frescos have been removed to the Museum of Naples for additional protection. There, suspended in the air of the colors on one panel, is the Dancer of Pompeii--or so I named her--carrying in one hand a disc, and in the other what might be the sceptre of the Dance itself. (In an issue of the Encylopedi Alpina, this figure is described as "Une bacchante portant le thyrse et l'oscillum").

I wondered who the artist had been who had chosen to decorate the walls of unpretentious domestic rooms with the very essence of the motions of Dance. I wondered how the beautiful colors of her robes had lasted through two thousand years. I wished that I might always come back to see her there, flanked by her dancing companions, telling the world of our time as she did of hers, that true Dance has always projected the spirit of man through the body of motion outward into space and time.

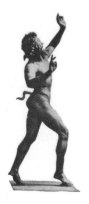

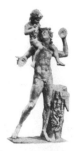

The Dancing Faun, originally marked the entrance to the Casa Fauna in Pompeii, now stands in the Naples Museum ... In the same museum is the statue described as "Faun carrying a Bacchus boy on its shoulders"

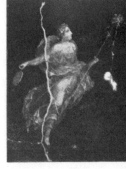 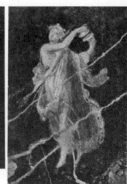 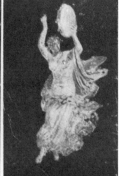

Bacchantes from Pompeiian frescoes, carrying sceptres, disks, cymbals and tambors. These frescoes have been removed to the National Museum at Naples to protect them against damage.

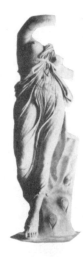

"The Dancer of Tivoli", a sculpture found in the National Museum in Rome, which, despite demolished head and arms, "... embodies the roundness and expansive breadth characteristic of the best in 'free' dance ..."

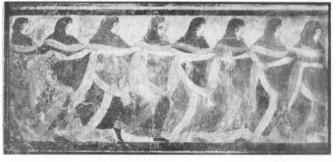

Ritual dance from the tombs of Rava, paintings whose colors of yellow, white, black, red and blue are remarkable preserved and three dimensional in effect.

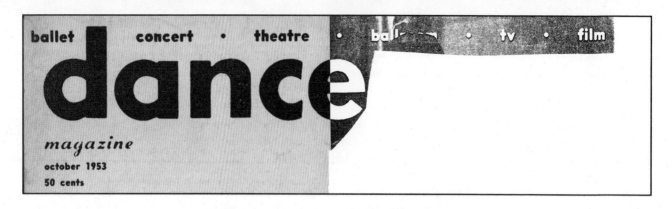

ballet · concert · theatre · ball---- · tv · film

dance

magazine

october 1953

50 cents

"I Always Wanted to Dance"
by Blanche Evan

Who "I" Am,
the first of a series of four articles — an exploration into the thoughts, dreams and problems of the amateur in modern dance.

Introduction

In the modern dance field, although there is occasional debate between exponents of dance in adult education and professional dance, almost no attention is given the amateur who dances once a week for reasons far removed from education per se.

I speak of the dance student who makes her living in the business world or who is a scholar or a housewife; who has no professional ambition but who "loves to dance" or has wanted to since childhood; or afraid to admit creative urges, thinks of dance study as "exercise" rather than as art. In recent years the once-a-week adult class has also included women who dance at the suggestion of their psychotherapists.

This series concerns itself with the adult amateur. It will outline her neglect by the American profession in terms of the factual evolution of dance in the United States, expound the layman's rightful position in dance activity , and suggest one kind of pedagogy that can yield the once-a-week student a measure of dignity and creative satisfaction.

The subject is vast and in these articles must be limited to some of the salient factors.

"I", to paraphrase *Ballad for Americans*, am the secretary, social worker, dental assistant, commercial artist, mother, housewife, stenographer, factory worker--I am Jeanne limp and sweet, tired from a day's work at school; I am Lini happily married and holding down a textile designer's job; and Sonia walking my feet off investigating social service needs. I am Clare, frustrated and fragile; and Freda, mother of two pre-school tots; and Eleanor with a son in high school. I am Rae burdened with a limp since my accident; and I am Frances and Rose and Mina, tense and lacking confidence, undergoing psychotherapy and advised by the analysts to dance.

For many years "I" postponed registering for dance class. Friends and family thought me ridiculous: ("dancing is for the stage...you have to start when you're a child...you have weak ankles and you're too skinny--or you're too fat...you're wasting your money", etc.); the dance profession thought me presumptuous and the dance critic lumped me with pathetic self-expression faddists. Most of all, "I" had myself to contend with: frustration, self-disparagement, my self-conscious ungainly body; my fear of exposure of physical weaknesses; my Puritan heritage of clamping down emotion: ("... the fear of emotional expression and the imprisonment of the personality in an unresponsive body...") (H'D).

The taunts of convention were partly true. "I" *was* no longer a child, but anywhere from 20 to 45, and I had hardly ever danced before except in my mind's eye, in my floating daydream and in my wish-fulfillment night dream wherein I could leap and stay in the air and land like a feather.

When Had My Dancing Dream Begun?

Freda:"...at the age of five...dancing to radio music...stopping dead with self-consciousness as the 'look-what-she's doing' attitude of the assembled adults penetrated. At six after some lessons I caught cold... immediately attributed by my elders to dancing in a drafty studio...lessons were terminated. At twelve and a half...by walking across town to High School instead of using the bus I had fifty cents a week for a clandestine class at the little local school. Dancing was the activity I craved more than any other..."

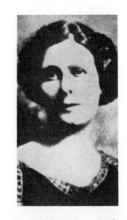

Isadora Duncan said of the dancer of the future: "She will dance the body emerging again from centuries of civilized forgetfulness."

Jeanne: "I had taken a year of dance lessons as a child and always a frustrated desire to continue them."

Lini: "Interested in physical exercise, I entered dancing school quite accidentally."

Eva: "I was quite young and I felt like a flower and a fairy also different types of seasonal climate!"

Eleanor:"...In my teens I had wanted to dance because I loved it. I was accepted at some big studio of ballet but my parents wouldn't let me go; they thought it might lead to stage work and then to them things theatrical were not real, not sound, too flip."

Rae: "I always longed to express myself artistically through the body. When I injured my hip that seemed the last straw in frustration. My analyst suggested functional and creative dance as adjunct to psychotherapy."

Clare:"...ever since I can remember I have wanted to dance...Being a thin rather sad, worrisome child mother refused me dancing lessons of any kind throughout childhood and adolescence. By then I was frustrated beyond words...but the desire was always there."

These particular students in my amateur class in creative dance had never attended a modern dance college, rarely a dance recital, nor had they heard of Diaghilev or Mary Wigman. They had wanted to dance *for its own inherent satisfactions*. They now study creative dance once weekly after work in group class much as other non-professionals engage in sculpture, painting or dramatics.

They speak for numbers of women in this country who have "always wanted to dance" and now are studying. They represent a new phenomenon in our culture; therefore it is important to sketch the background that helped produce amateur dance in our time and country.

Freedom

The American adult traditionally has been physically repressed--a victim of "...the rigidity and ritual of our national religion of negation..."(XE). The "free" social dances at the turn of the century set a new and raucous note and were avidly adopted: in 1900 the turkey-trot; 1910, the sensuous tango; 1912, the foxtrot followed by the shimmy, the Charleston, and in 1926 the Black Bottom.

At the turn of the century the art of dance had barely reached the public. Havelock Ellis wrote:"... those of us who still appreciated dancing as an art--and how few there were!--had to seek for it painfully and sometimes in strange surroundings". Soon after 1900 America produced three shining stars in the art dance: Loie Fuller with her sensational use of light and color; Ruth St. Denis theatrically inclined and a devotee of the Eastern dance; and Isadora Duncan who though inspired by both ancient Greek dance and by the best of classical music, nevertheless danced essentially her own new found freedom through an emancipated body. She was the forerunner of our whole history of dance as an individual expression.

Duncan was known to end many a recital with diatribes on the inhibitions of the American woman but in her school her desire was "to teach the children and the youth."(ID) St. Denis concentrated on adults.

Both artists helped to break down the outer walls of prejudice. However the active resurgence of dance *as an expressive art for the layman* occurred not here but in Germany in post World War I. Led by Laban and Wigman, the German dance brought into focus *the difference between the professional and the amateur* and, with no loss to their professional integrity, held the amateur in such high regard as to develop the "group dance chorus". Certain German schools, Bode for instance, existed solely for layman. The Wigman curriculum formulated distinct phases of dance entirely new in Western Dance pedagogy: "gymnastics, dance gymnastics, group dance, improvisation, composition, percussion, history of dance music, pedagogy and related subjects." Education *for* dancing involved the "strengthening, clarifying and intensifying of the creative impulses..."(VS:M)

Duncan had had so much conviction in spontaneity as to improvise for Carnegie Hall audiences. She valued, unashamedly, *inspiration* and *freedom of expression*. The beneficent influence of the new German dance also had seeped into America. In both, technique had been regarded as preparation *for* dance not as an end in itself. Above and beyond technique stood improvisation, a separate and highly esteemed branch of experience.

Both Duncan and Wigman performed an impressive recital repertoire. Their free approach did not lessen their consciousness of form. Though worlds apart in other ways, both believed that each dance demanded fresh movement images derived from its specific content, from total experience and individual attributes. Composition grew out of the fluidity of improvisation and was unrestricted by past or present academic molds.

THIS APPROACH AS A WHOLE WAS CONDUCIVE TO CREATIVE PARTICIPATION BY THE LAYMAN.

Why then despite these propelling forces of freedom was the amateur hard put to find an American school in which the stress was on the individual? After 25 years, dance for the layman is still the stepchild of our profession. The inexperienced adult is compelled for the most part to enter classes of professional dance limited to formal approaches in technique and composition.

THE AMERICAN MODERN DANCE HAD BECOME ACADEMIC WITHIN ITS OWN EXPERIMENTATIONS.

Formalism

From 1925 on, the leading American professional modern dancers cut ties with the artistic concepts of their immediate predecessors and developed in extremely opposite direction. The new drive was *away from* "freedom" and "expression" toward theatricalism and formalism. They did succeed in creating a disciplined branch of the profession and in the process ruled out a place for the amateur. The Denishawn dissidents: Graham, Humphrey, Weidman and Horst, each sought an individualistic theory as a basis for the new dance--something that would be typical of America. Each innovator emerged with a new "technique" dictated by somewhat abstruse theory, heavily marked by mannerism and personal style, upon which were grafted borrowed forms. (Composer

Arnold Schonberg deplores a similar trend in modern music. "Today the majority strives for style, technique and sound; meaning thereby something purely external" (AScA).

STYLISTIC TECHNIQUE BECAME THE DOMINATING CHARACTERISTIC OF THE NEW AMERICAN MODERN DANCE. ITS PURPOSE WAS TO DEVELOP STUDENT PERFORMERS FOR PROFESSIONAL RECITAL APPEARANCE.

The technique thus devised lacked impersonality and employed extreme uses of the body. It trained students in a mannered skill becoming a trademark of the choreographer until there was little movement differentiation between class technique and movements arbitrarily employed in composition. To have imitators is one thing. To create them is another. The creation of miniature replicas of the leaders of the American modern dance by the leaders themselves led to robots cluttering the solo recital stages and the gyms of almost every college where dance is offered. As the leaders later broadened their scope they left a pitiful trail behind them of all the lambs that had submissively, in awe and in fright, followed them to school.

Improvisation became outmoded. Form no longer evolved primarily out of content. A dance took shape by reference to musical and poetical forms: ABA, Theme and Variations, Fugue, etc.; and by reference to the austere, patterned pre-classic dance forms: pavane, minuet, sarabande, etc. of the conventional 18th century. These forms contributed knowledge and historical background but they lacked spiritual connection with the modern dance of the 20th century. (The modern dance repertoire contains great works illuminated by their formal structure but this should not rule out improvisational approaches to choreography. As an individualistic branch of dance a liquid compositional form may yet be its most effective channel for creation.)

This approach as a whole could not admit of dancing as transient pleasure. The amateur student had no chance "to dance" except as a member of a performing group. Since most amateurs could not devote time sufficient to admit them into performing groups, their activity narrowed down solely to technique. The layman was swept into this whirlpool of professional purpose although denied the satisfactions of adequate training. Furthermore she herself did not wish to be professional and lacked the equipment for the profession. Her ambition was not to perform nor primarily to execute another's choreography.

The opportunity came with the second generation of American modern dancers. They needed large groups to realize their choreographic ambitions when the WPA projects opened up opportunities for unemployed dancer-choreographers; the political left movement, in the upsurge of the time, stressed amateur group performances (even holding contests on dances of contemporary social themes). Recital dancers, relying on teaching for a living (as in all arts) to absorb their deficit-yielding concerts, began to realize the potential of this newly-found amateur student body. (Today, after twenty years, even the die-hard professional ballet schools include "classes for the business girls" in their curricula.)

Let Her Again Speak for Herself

"I" who had "always wanted to dance" was now at last in a dance studio. But, my body was treated like a exalted machine and my dream of using the body to express myself found no realization. I looked around me. These professionals did not seem to need "to dance". Perhaps for them that would come later. They burned with ambition, perseverance; they were dogged in their determination to acquire that super-skill necessary for competition in performance, none of which was part of my world at all.

"I" ached with unnatural pain from the distortions for which my body was physically unprepared. My knees swelled. The vocabulary was mysterious. And I could find little connection between my one class hour and my body of day-to-day living.

"I" still wanted to dance. I read with envy of amateur dance in Spain, where the working girl danced every night for hours as part of her cultural heritage:

"In the evening it is warm and there is a moon. A dozen pairs of castanuelas are sounding...guitars tune up in the corner. Fifteen or so girls of all ages move about the room...while their parents sit on the wooden benches against the wall. The girls are in street dresses. They have come here straight from their work, for they are stenographers, salesgirls, tobacco-factory workers, seamstresses. They dance because they love it; because they are Andalucian. Every night they come for two or three hours...and any fiesta, public or private, is graced by their dancing...Near midnight the girls reluctantly break it up out of respect for their workaday tomorrow. This happens every night, but no one ever gets tired of it, for this is Seville."(LaM)

But this is not Seville. This is New York; and this is America. In the professional approaches, many layman were hurt physiologically and emotionally. Many gave up all hope of dance as a creative activity, they discontinued, disillusioned and empty.

THE PROBLEM IS NOT TO MINIMIZE PROFESSIONAL STANDARDS BUT TO FIND AN ORIENTATION FOR THE AMATEUR.

Teachers here and there have worked quietly behind the scenes for many years. Their results more than confirm the idea that there is a place and need for amateur participation in dance as a "means of enjoying and enriching life through *creative* experience".(VD'A)

Bibliography

AScA: Arnold Schonberg in *Schonberg* edited by Armitage (also see: *Modern Composers* by Ewen; *Style and Idea* by *Schonberg*

ID: Isadora Duncan: The Art of Dance

LaM: La Meri: Spanish Dancing

H'D: Mgt. H'Doubler: The Dance:A Creative Art Experience

VD'A: Victor D'Amico: Creative Teaching in Art

VS:M Michael in Virginia Stewart's *Modern Dance*

XE: Max Eastman: in Havelock Ellis' *The Dance of Life also:* F.R. Rogers (edit): *Dance: A Basic Educational Technique* Hans Sachs: *The Creative Unconscious* ballet • concert • theatre • ballroom • tv • film

dance

magazine

november 1953

50 cents

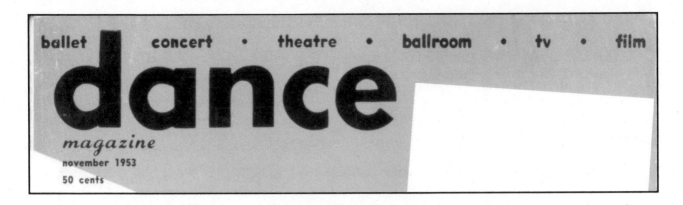

"I Always Wanted to Dance"
by Blanche Evan

II. The Artist and the Amateur

"I" register for a course in Creative Dance

> I: *An imaginary composite of actual students*

> R. *Registrar*

"I". (At last...here I am... after years...years)

R. Come in--can I help you?

"I". Yes--I'd like to inquire about your courses. (*Why have I delayed?...extreme shyness--protection against my own anxieties--fear of professional dance schools; my age, too--Then marriage and children...only three weeks my second child was born. I've dreamed of this day...my heart is pounding*).

R. Have you ever danced before?

"I". When I was a kid I had a few lessons (*and clinging still to their memory. Those long Friday nights when I never slept a wink waiting for Saturday--that was dancing day...the thrill of moving gracefully in class--the once each week I crawled out of my shell. The world became beautiful*).

R. What form of dance do you wish to study?

"I". Well--I don't exactly know what it's called..modern ballet, I think.

R. There's no such thing as "modern ballet". We do teach a course in Classical Ballet fundamentals but our main work is in Creative Dance.

"I". What do you do in creative dance? (*Could this be it? to make my body speak for me--all the pent up emotion...and as if she read my thoughts--*)

R. Creative Dance, like all true art, expresses yourself. I know what you're thinking: how can you express yourself through your body when you don't know *how* to dance...

"I". (My body--this tense clumsy flabby wobbly thing...I've watched it change with consternation, and become what it is through these difficult years.)

R.   Of course we teach you how. But technique should be used only as a means to an end. If you came week in and week out to do only technique, as is done in many studios, it would be like forever oiling up a motor car that never left the garage to take you anywhere.

For us the technique is functional: restoring nature's unmatched mechanisms: posture alignment; strengthening long unused muscles, relaxing the wrongly used...

"I". I don"t understand. That doesn't sound like dancing.

R.   The technique helps transform your body into an instrument *for* dance. As a child nobody had to tell you to jump for joy or retract with fear--your body just had to. You must work your way back to that state of spontaneity wherein the body is no stranger to your emotions but a direct outlet of them and of your imagination. This is the objective of dance improvisation as we use it and it begins in your very first lessons.

"I". Do we ever learn a finished dance?

R.   (*Interesting that she skips over this matter of improvisation--doesn't ask a thing about it--she must already be frightened of the idea.*) Yes, occasionally an authentic folk dance.

"I". Do we ever make up our own dances?

R.   "Form" comes much later.   First we gain the ability to improvise; later we compose.

"I". But once a week. How can we do all that?

R.   A good question. Only by planned pedagogy on the teacher's part and by the keenest mental--muscular application on your own. And over many, many seasons. Not a moment is wasted. The classroom atmosphere is just as intense as that for professionals.

"I". The dancing you describe sounds like an art and I'm no dancer--I never will be.

R.   I do expect of amateurs something of the dedication of their class work that professionals must give during a whole life time.

"I". This worries me. Please explain.

R.   The axis of all true art, whether produced by professionals or amateurs, is the expression of the individual's reactions to the world in which he lives.

This is the first of the ties between the amateur and the artist: who"...portrays himself...and that which therefore would remain inaccessible to anyone else..."(ACcS) (his--the artist's--main source is his Unconscious and he finds the pattern...in himself") (HS).

Much of your work here will be to plummet and dig to bring out, in dance, that expressive self which is now submerged but potentially vital. This process, as a catharsis for ambitions, constitutes an objective in dance therapy; in the study of creative dance, by laymen particularly, it is a necessary step to creation, but only one step. When you have lifted yourself over it, you are more ready to use the materials of dance and may, like the artist,"...attain beauty without willing it"(ASc).

"I". I really don't feel worthy...one year I try painting, then music, now dancing--

R.   You like thousands of others have felt the need to find a place, to express your relation to the world. An amateur is apt to try one art after another in search of that one that yields her satisfaction. By contrast the artist's desire exists from the beginning, fused with the need to create mainly in a *chosen* art--chosen by nature and given as an unborn gift.

Another reason for frequent shifting is that an amateur will cease the activity if its pain should exceed its pleasure. To the artist pain and pleasure are not the issue; what matters is to be active and to create in terms of his art.

The amateur can experience art best by *active participation*--a far cry from the rather barren, "art appreciation" courses flooding educational curricula. Here you will become involved with "...the sheer joy of handling materials" (HC); without which you can only gaze upon art with a limited (even though absorbing) response...With the help of authentic music and literary references we also introduce you to dance of other kinds and cultures to help you conceive of dance as a universal art experience.

This quest for knowledge of the fabric of an art in its physical and philosophical aspects constitutes the second great binder between the dance artist and amateur.

"I".   Do you mean "I" won't be looking on from the outside any longer?

R.   Why should you be?

"I".   According to you anyone, if he tries hard enough, can be an artist?

R.   That idea is prevalent today and of course it depends on definition. I myself feel that talent either is or is not inborn. No pedagogy can create it but it can discover it and develop it.

"I".   What about those of us who don't show talent?

R.   Our purpose is not to mold artists but to lead you to experience the art of dance in its basic phases.

"I".   But even a talented layman is far from being an artist.

R.   And one of the main differences is that the layman lives in the dance-as-art sporadically whereas the artist must live in its intensity relentlessly--must and wants to and is unhappy if she cannot:"...to live in the world of creation--to get into it--to frequent it and haunt it".(HJ);...But for now it is more important to accept the basic affinities.

After several seasons, you will develop such an eye inward and outward for honest movement it will be difficult to fool you. You run the risk of becoming a snob--not in favor of the arty, but of the true; not seeking virtuosity but essence; not the externally theatrical but the deeply profound. By the way none of this excludes the humorous except that it is uncommon to find convincing comedy in dance. Charles Weidman and Lotte Goslar have been exceptional in this respect.

"I".   Can I register for just a few lessons to see if I like it? (*Like it! Suppose I'm too self-conscious to come back.*)

R.   No, we don't work that way. The adjustment may take a full term. Be patient and remember that the class is geared to you, to the kind of amateur I have described. Those who wish only to exercise; those who want *to copy* rather than *to become*--they drop out soon enough.

"I".   Have the others danced before?

R.   You really mean, don't you, that you feel dreadfully timid? Each member of the class suffers some measure of fright and uneasiness and self-consciousness...

"I".   (How does she know...she must have had hundreds like me...)

R.   ...but each is too self-concerned to pay you any attention. But you are not alone in your negative approaches. As of our modern psychiatrist says: "The great majority of us have to struggle with problems of competition, fears of failure, emotional isolation, distrust...of our own selves...produced by the difficulties existing in our time and culture".(KH)

No...twelve lessons is a minimum, taken in successive weeks, and with absences made up.

"I".   Will it help to practise at home? (*I can just see the grin on my husband's face*).

R.   Improvise yes. Few people practise technique at home--professionals themselves prefer a class. Besides, the technique should be part of your body throughout the working day and not at a "set-aside" twenty minute practise time.

"I".   Like what?

R.   To "sit vertically" at your desk; arches pulled up within your shoes; balancing in the subway without holding the strap, running for the bus with breath--that is running *on* the ground instead of pounding *into* it--walking with a lifted head and with stomach muscles actively pulling inward...

"I".   (*How exciting--and nobody around me will even know I'm "practising"*)

R.   Living body architecture will be more valuable at first than "exercises". It constitutes exercise in itself--(muscles uphold as well as move bones)--and it becomes an important means of transforming your negative concept of your own body.

"I".   How will I ever get to work the day after class!

R.   As a matter of fact,you will rarely be exhausted at the end of class--not for many weeks until you learn *how* to work, in which time you will be building your endurance. The exercises are not the "knock you out" kind. They will be graded starting at the level of your power.   But--one thing--at first you do not know your own power.   Your teacher may make demands upon you that seem beyond it. Here you must trust her insight and experience. You can progress beyond your present potential only if *the measure of power as it now exists in you is used to the full*. The standard is your best body.

"I".   Are the classes crowded?

R.   No--the pedagogy was created with the individual student in mind. Besides, the number of adults willing to concentrate so deeply and to wait for results, is limited. After all, once a week--time, time, and more time is what counts.

"I".   When I come to class next week, what shall I wear?

R.   Anything in which you feel comfortable.

"I".   Thank you...Before I go, may I ask how come that you as a professional have given so much time and thought to the cause of the layman?

R.   Let me say at first that despite its merciless demands were I to choose all over again it would be to be a dancer; nothing in the world has ever been more beautiful to me....Perhaps it was unconsciously to satisfy some need of attachment to the social scene--the orbit of the creative dance soloist has been so limited--and to widen the horizon of creative dance itself. It has worked out in unexpected ways: for example Sheila, who came to study with me as a child of eleven, now an assistant teacher here, is at present taking her Master's Degree at Columbia in the almost untouched field of dance therapy as part of rehabilitation. With the kind of dance foundation we have discussed many students continue to dance non-professionally simply because they love it. Others become professional dancers and choreographers.

Incidentally it was only because of the depth and uncompromising intensity of my professional outlook that I have been able to draw out the essence for the amateur.

"T". Your last point reassures me. I wish other laymen could know that art and amateur work can be truly related. *I always wanted to dance* but until to-night I never knew I had the right.

BIBLIOGRAPHY

ASc: Arnold Schonberg in *Modern Composers* by Ewen

AScS: Arnold Schonberg: *Style and Idea* by Schonberg

HC: Henry Caudwell: *The Creative Impulse*

HJ: Henry James in HC

HS: Hans Sachs: *The Creative Unconscious*

KH: Katherine Horney: *The Neurotic Personality of Our Time*

Z: William Zorach: *Zorach Explains Sculpture*

photos by darwin

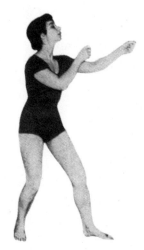 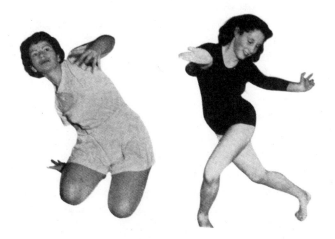

L. to R.: Jean, Sonia and Wendy improvise on themes of "fishing", "time on a binge" and "losing and finding".

"T", to paraphrase *Ballad for Americans*, am the secretary, social worker, dental assistant, commercial artist, mother, housewife, stenographer, factory worker . . .

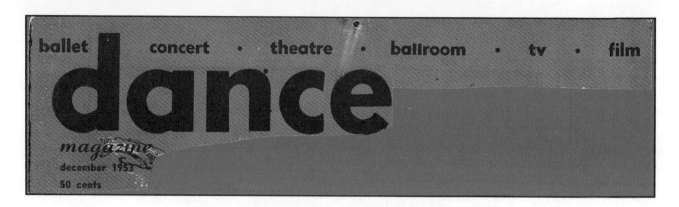

ballet · concert · theatre · ballroom · tv · film

dance
magazine
december 1953
50 cents

"I Always Wanted to Dance"
by Blanche Evan

III. The Miracle of Myself

We continue to seek a basic a technique for creative dance that will respect the body's limitations and at the same time establish a comprehensive base for movement potential. It is clear that we must be governed by such knowledge as we can obtain of the function and structure of the body. Man constructed the instruments of the other arts but in the case of dance (and voice) the instrument was constructed for him. "Human ingenuity" can never devise anything more simple and more beautiful or to the purpose than Nature does", according to the wise words of Leonardo De Vinci. The creation and selection of a dance technique plain and undramatic, devoid of pat "forms" of expression, can leave the student relatively free of influence, and make the way clear for the student's own movement imagery.

The "I" who "always wanted to dance" may be a woman of 20 or 30 or even 40 years, with body set in a lifetime of physical habits: Drooping shoulders, lax stomach muscles, feet conditioned by the high-heeled shoe--hips thrust back in sway-back, etc. This body must be prepared for dance. We should set about to undo the misalignments; to transfer the energy of muscles acting under nervous tension and to build up muscles to support the new alignment to its proper function. Alignment refers, of course, to posture. To the layman, posture is located mostly in "spots": "I have round shoulders", or "my hips stick out". One of the most difficult pedagogic tasks is to convince her that posture is the result of the reconditioning of the entire body--balancing the relationship of one part to another--not a place. For instance, reconstruction of the shoulders is of little avail if the feet are weak and unable to support the body. Conversely, a new stance will change the tonicity of the feet. "Good posture" may be the last achievement after seasons of work.

The dancer has to contend directly and indirectly with the four hundred and thirty four muscles and two hundred and six bones of the body--it is clear that without a postural center, she would be lost. The dancer's objective is to achieve a basic stance from which she can deviate far in movement, but with security, since she can return to it through conscious control. Postural attainment for daily carriage can be treated as an isolated objective only in the very first phase of correcting misalignment. Beyond that, the use of posture in dance makes demands upon it not essential to its limited through magnificient everyday use.

There are some of the concepts that need revision in the attitudes of the amateur. And then there are the many concepts to be born. Let the student address you in her own terms.

"I" Speaks:

I am now in a studio where I am compelled to see myself as I am--horrible thought! For instance I was asked to observe how the joints of my toes move. Probably for the first time since infancy, I really looked at my feet--and I was so fascinated at their movement I found myself taking off my socks (I was the only one in the class wearing them). I no longer saw the malformations and the ugly corn--I saw the toes and ankles go up, down, pointing one up, the other down, finally each ankle describing a circle.

We learned the six basic directions; forward, back, side, up, down, and their connecting vertical and horizontal circles, and applied them to action of the joints separately and in their unified deportment. "Exercises of Discovery" they were to me. It is intriguing that each shoulder is constructed to move independently on the shoulder girdle, but that where one hip goes, the other has to follow! When asked to curve my spine forward to the ground and move my back up and down I "naturally" bounce my head thinking--erroneously--it is my back!

When I stretch forward I make a great effort but the harder I try the more my muscles tighten and the less I can "reach". There is so much to understand.

The Teacher Explains:

When you stretch forward, the front muscles contract while those along the back need to lengthen. If, instead, you contract them through nervous or misplaced effort, you prevent them from stretching. Obviously you cannot make a rubber band long and short simultaneously; a muscle behaves similarly. You can add intensity to a stretching muscle beyond functional necessity, but that becomes dramatic and is out of place in these fundamentals.

Your body now is full of forced and false contractions acquired through disuse; through careless habits of movement, and produced by mental tensions. Together they add up to muscular rigidity. The unnecessary muscular contractions act like rivets of petrified wood blocking the natural spring or leverage of the body. Frozen muscles and petrified joints prevent both stretch and spring; they make impossible the functioning of allotted muscles for their work; they prevent the employment of muscles as expressive vehicles of dramatic or emotional content. They can be dangerous since they interfere with the body's reflexes of self-protection.

We cannot here remove the emotional causes of your tensions--that is within the role of psychiatry, not of dance. But we can temper the nervous effort and try to remove the misplaced muscular tensions that interfere with function; reduce them to a state of relaxation so that they may take on their true functions; and redirect all this wasted energy to purposeful expenditure.

"I":

This new attitude toward my muscles brings tangible results whereas the constant advice of a dancing friend to "relax", had been to no avail. Our aim is getting clear to me. It's to achieve maximum power with minimum strain.

We do no extreme movements; these basic exercises, with their logical growth in complexity, are difficult to do meticulously, for they seem to tap the very roots of function. Each new movement is a surprise, yet fits into the whole like a spoke in a wheel.

As the weeks go by I find I no longer resent my body. The revelation of the powers given by nature and now being restored, disclose a miracle of structure and purpose--the miracle of myself. My body has been a treasure chest with the locked turn rusty and I have been so ignorant of its wonders. I am relieved of the burden of emulating the ideal professional dancer's body--I understand and accept the fact that my body is the instrument for expressing *me*.

Yes, first to restore. It is not easy, but even at my age muscles can respond and my body can cope with dance problems of coordination and balance. As for balance, I sometimes wonder why we are so afraid of it (*Does it symbolize the core of our insecurity?*)

Teacher:

The child learns to walk by stumbling as well as by standing straight. Isn't it more interesting to lose your balance dancing than not to lose it in a safe position? Balance is learning to make the continuous, linked adjustments to center. Though balance appears to be still, it is the least static of all dance phenomena: like a placid sea that holds beneath its surface all its turbulent life and shifting currents.

"I":

Our lessons begin to move more and more from the realm of functional exercise to dance technique and rhythmic improvisations. At times we do kid-stuff--walking, and simple elevations; how embarrassing that I didn't know how to gallop. We did swing coordinations and waltz rhythms--the latter surprisingly difficult since the waltz is to be in the body rather than in feet first.

It was many many weeks later when we were asked to improvise--no, not on "Voices of Spring"--but on:

Lead Belly Work Songs!

"What should we do?" We had learned nothing in our so-called technique that we could use to express the song. Eighteen lessons and we had no mold in which to shape a dance...no technical form to be used as a shell for expression.

We listened to the music and analyzed the words--hammers and picking cotton and the frenzy indicated by the singer--and how frenzy might make for disorder in one's space directions or it might make one stick rigidly to a fixed line of direction. Best of all I was not asked to "express" myself. That would have been utterly embarrassing and at this stage, fruitless. I didn't mind, perhaps I was even eager, to put myself in the place of someone in the outside world.

Soon the room was transformed into dance. That music was too definite in beat and too compelling for us to just mime the words. We were exhausted. And then the flood of questions; "Is that what you wanted?" we asked the teacher.

"I wanted only for you to dance as you felt."

"But is what we did right?"

And her answer: "Was it right for you?" (*no satisfaction here*).

"Well, I enjoyed it!"

"Then isn't that enough for your first improvisation on a work theme?"

"But I don't remember what I did."

"That," she said as she put the disc away, "is because you enjoyed it." (*I didn't understand until two seasons later what the teacher really meant: to lose one's self in improvisation is to find a deeper self.*)

Strange Pulls:

In the fifth lesson of the third season, about the 77th hour of study, we delved into the strangest class we had ever had. Did you ever place your right leg into a back left diagonal lift, with arms held, your right arm away in a downward right diagonal and the left straight forward? And use such a design in moving through space by changing locomotion? (*Is this sheer perversity to confuse us?*) So the lesson went--mathematically; its purpose to "disassociate" our limbs--later the torso, too-- from that very ease of direction we had worked so hard to attain. A series was then built which the teacher called a "Study." It reminded me of the pianistic studies of Clementi and Czerny in that it was "developed on a single theme and designed to perfect the student in a certain mechanical problem." We were not permitted to call it a dance. Its sole purpose was experience and practice in "disassociation."

We were then asked to take supine positions to start with, thus making it impossible to repeat the movements we had learned. The strangest music I had ever heard filled the room. "This improvisation will be called "Strange Pulls."

Our bodies succeeded in breaking the patterns of symmetry and habits of movement though these habits now looked *good*: that is they were no longer careless, they spoke of acquired skill not made automatic. We had reached a point where it was necessary to inform us, always through action, of the range of movement happily known to dance, in order to have at our command growing technical scope for growing content.

Exploration had now advanced from the miracle of myself to the miracle of the movement of dance.

Riding home in the subway that night I remembered--it came to me in a flash--the time when once before I had tried to improvise on a theme called "asymmetry", and failed. I had forgotten all about it. Though it had been meant for me I had dropped it by the wayside on the heap of unfinished experience. No wonder the teacher's class notes are so thick--filled with lost thoughts of so many students, and with ways to follow up their tracks and so establish continuity despite the limitations of once-a-week class.

(*The final article of this series appears in the January issue*) ballet · concert · theatre · ballroom · tv · film

dance

magazine

january 1954

50 cents

"I Always Wanted to Dance"

by Blanche Evan

"The Terror of Myself"
The 4th and Final article of a series on the Amateur in the Dance.

INTRODUCTION

Block, barrier, obstacle--these are the word images that come to mind as I recall many students in their first improvisations. Clinging to the wall, stopping as if dead in the middle of movement, the face assuming a semi-mask appearance to hide the depths of embarrassment and the feelings of inadequacy.

WHY did "I" always want to dance?

How painful it must be to want to express an emotion, even a simple rhythm or mood through one's body and yet feel prevented from within. The teacher's work lies not in probing into the causes of the students' resistance, but rather in devising methods for transmuting terror to self-confidence, dissolving blockades between desire and its realization. There are pedagogic devices for "disarming the resistance" (HS) and for "dissipating apprehensions" (F:W); and methods for stimulating the imagination, for changing habit to newness in movement. These are ways "to increase the force available for application to work" and means "for transmitting power from the engine shaft to the driving wheels" (W)--the ongoing wheels of the student herself.   B.E.

THE STUDENTS HOLD A ROUND TABLE DISCUSSION

RAE: A friend of mine wanted to register here for a class in "exercise." It seems she was tactfully advised to go to a good gym. She was told that dance is an art, an expressive medium, and that every course includes basic work in creative dance. I wonder how many of us expected to do creative work in our first season?

CLARE: I didn't--not at all...I thought that was only for professionals. And how surprised I was to find myself doing simple creative things before I realized it...

FREDA: I expected to improvise right from the beginning. "Creative work" sounds like a larger, grander thing than applies to me now. I'm not interested at this time in creating a dance as an end in itself so much as I am in the doing of it--in the using myself more fully.

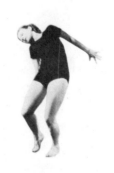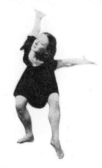

RAE: Improvisation can do that more than any other kind of dance activity, I think, even though it takes longer to "get into it".

ELEANOR: It took me a full season, but in those few instances when I really expressed something in dance, I got a big thrill. This year I actually contributed to our group composition. The first year I was terribly ashamed to move, much less compose, in the presence of others.

JEAN: It's a good idea not to have anyone observe our classes. No one watching could understand our self-consciousness. Because we don't have mastery over our bodies we feel self-conscious; then the self-consciousness further inhibits movement, causing a vicious circle.

MINA: It's not just lack of technical mastery...perhaps we're ashamed that we're not beautiful--we won't take a chance on calling forth unflattering comparisons. But then, our improvisations are rarely criticized...perhaps we can't bear even self-criticism.

JEAN: Whatever it is, I do believe that to relax emotionally-physically and to overcome self-consciousness are essential to creative expression, particularly in dance, where muscles freeze up under mental tension.

("Beauty and anxiety can never dwell together") (HS)

CLARE: I've been dreadfully self-conscious in everything, dancing included,--but when the students in class didn't watch me improvise--even teacher purposely left the room at times--it subsided. Then it was completely gone in class and instead I've had a new feeling of freedom I've been able to take with me outside of class. (Inferiority subsides, the sense of phantom staring eyes directed critically to me, recedes.)

RAE: You mean self-expression is not a negative escape...

CLARE: I've danced out so much that was otherwise held in, including the feeling of unkindness that is in all of us...Depression comes less frequently and stays for shorter intervals, giving me a chance to breathe, to broaden my outlook on life, to take an interest in others, understand them when their feeling and moods can't be released...I began to like being with people...I'm a different person altogether...

ROSE: The dance as you experienced it helped you almost directly to face reality.

FREDA: Self-consciousness still hampers me a good deal. I'm mildly uncomfortable improvising before others, but what is more important. I am self-conscious *with myself* so that I am limited in the ways I move completely apart from an audience.

MINA: "Self-consciousness with myself"--with that astute comment Freda takes away our last self-deception!

ROSE: I just can't break the ice. I *always* have a theatre date or meeting--liar me--I *must* leave as soon as technique stops and creative work begins. I just sidle over to the door quietly but purposefully.

RAE: And I make as if to stay but slip out unnoticed, or so I hope--Anyone would think we didn't *want* to do creative work...

LINI: It seems a long time ago...I felt very inhibited about doing anything in class...I remember...in my first improvisation...I was panic stricken...

("His confidence shall be rooted out...and it shall bring him to the king of terrors") (J)

Terror has many faces. Laughter is one of them--there is always one student who giggles her way through her first dozen lessons. Resentment is another: "It's interesting this, but I came for exercise." Plebianism is another: "This concentration in sacred silence gets me. Why not get down to earth!" "Earth" here means the fatuous, the superficial play, the whispered gossip. Or, "When do we study composition or learn some dances?"-- a wish to be handed a ready made feast of other people's choreographic dishes, or the desire to hide vacuity in the comforting formulae of form: of ABA and Theme and Variation, etc. Clothed in discontent of one kind or another, these students really point up their inability to tread through the pressure of that silence in which each must be faced with all her suppressed desire to express herself--for who among them does not wish this? They come to the art of their own volition and yet are ashamed.

Improvisation is most effective for dispelling the very inner terror its contemplation sometimes generates; for in improvisation one idea takes precedence over the scattered and confused self--and absorbs it. The theme, the thing to be expressed, becomes more important than the "I" of every day and, in a sense, takes possession of the body; so that by concentration and deep involvement with one's theme can achieve an "active performance under one's own power". (CS)

The spirit, the idea, the content commands, and the body executes. The spirit is wise, and perhaps because at such times it is indivisible with the body, its technical demands on the body seldom overreach the body's immediate aptitudes.

Freed from the sense of inferiority and the strictures of self-consciousness, without sentimentality and artifice, one can release the energy usually expended on maintaining attitudes rather than truths. Utilising the sweet unity of a self no longer divided, one spontaneously creates movement that is often complex and artistic.

When an improvisation is finished, there is no shame for having released an inhibition even when the material of the dance has been of a personal nature. Creative energy has transformed the "undisclosed, voiceless, and shapeless emotions" (HS) into an immediate form: A dance has taken shape with body, mind and spirit integrated in rare unity. The dancing person is left with a sense of completion and of release from the echoes of persistent wailing of our inner selves.

"Terrors shall make him afraid on every side"--yes--but they shall also "drive him to his feet". (J)

"His feet are set on the path...of beauty, but it needs something more than that to reach the stage of its actual evocation". (HS)

Self expression in dance is not an emotional state. Let us not confuse the heightened feeling necessary for its production with the action which it produces. Self-expression in dance is the transmutation of emotion into motion. It is the activity of dance in a poetic form, a rhythmic-spatial form different from composition but no less a form.

The "emotional reality" which forms the base of real improvisation, real spontaneity, "has nothing to do with the realistic or naturalistic rendering of emotion...motion...its freedom...that is, its irresponsibility and irregularity, is brought under the domination of unformulated but none the less strict rules...some of them unknown...demanding various forms of retardation, repetition, and other restrictions and regulations of the emotional outflow". (HS) Some of these elements of control are in the confinement of space, the body's self-protection from danger in movement. the natural tides and span of intensity, and, of uppermost importance, the limitations imposed by the content itself.

"For pure feeling could be expressed only in unorganized sounds, colours or lines; it would create a shriek, a daub or a scribble; while pure thought could lead only to some form of expression approximating mathematics. All art lies between the two extremes of feeling and thought and consists of a blend of the two". (HO)

In improvisation the state of involvement is far removed as well from the transcendence of the "ecstatic" dancer of certain primitive cultures and of some Eastern dances.

In our dancing, thought plays its part, but it is thought led by the silent hand of spirit, of knowledge, and of the expression of deep self through the channels of dance movement.

WHAT THE STUDENTS DANCE ABOUT

Things desired but forgotten, things remembered and imagined, of real memory and imagined memory, of to-day and of to-morrow,--clothed in terms of mood, dynamic description of specific ideas. Though one can never divine a dance from its title, these lists of student themes from one of the classes are of interest: For improvisation--gay (jazz); primitive drums; Latin American rhythms; relaxation; blues; violent, raucous; very slow, very big; time on a binge; gladness in the rain. Themes for composition among the same students included--From fall to flight; "Dream and its distortion in reality" (Kipling); southern slave wants freedom; question mark; pendulum; to want and to have not; conflict; my cycles; soothing.

The students were brought face to face with their resistance to honest expression by being assigned these themes: "Solitude", "Study of Me" and "Shriek". The theme of "Me" was broken down to separate improvisations: shy, aggressive, arrogant, dainty, vulgar, etc. By asking the student to indicate what percussion accompaniment they wished for the studies of "Me", they were further helped toward clarity.

For "Shriek"--in terms of movement, not voice--sometimes the improvisations were done to specially selected recordings, sometimes in silence. One of the students with many years of improvisations behind her, nevertheless refused at all times to participate in this.

To attain contrasting values, the themes presented by the teacher in other lessons were almost slight: ("the surface is the uppermost plane but it can mirror the depths") (TR): March, Bear, Mechanical Doll, Waltz, etc., from Shostakovich's Children's Suite. The adults loved the stimulation and recall value offered in the images used in children's play.

To help the students experience the freedom of movement known to more exotic cultures than ours, we used Hawaiian chants one evening; and while practising hip rotations, one student commented "this makes me feel wonderful" but later changed the response to "I feel demoralized".

Self-exploration is important. So also is dancing with others. In this group, simple partner improvisations and group dances on folk themes some taught to the group, others composed by the class, were effective controls over self-indulgence and helped the students reach out into positive social feelings in dance.

It is not possible to include here pedagogic methods for teaching the processes of improvisation; nevertheless it is clear that the student is not and should not be left to wander aimlessly within her emotional sphere, nor to seek oblivion in the accompaniment used. Nor can I here include the methods for making the transition from improvisation to composition.

Improvisation requires learning and experience no less than does body technique: to widen the imagination, to train it to function spontaneously, to train the body to reflect the wish, and the mind to produce the content appropriate for the medium of body movement. All this takes time but given time even the "untalented" eventually produce dance that is true, communicative, and often inspiring. (BE)

CONCLUSION

To accept the ideas proposed in this series one must agree that in our time there is necessary a renewed regard for the "common" and complex emotions of people and a new respect for the individual's right and need to express them in terms of amateur art; and that the work produced can be of high calibre. Such insistence on the "I" is frank recognition that to contribute best to the social good the "I" must find fulfillment in personal ways.

Havelock Ellis wrote of dance not only as "the supreme manifestation of physical life" (HE). The dance suffers in our times from an overdose of the physical with its emphasis on virtuosity and technical invention. It becomes additionally removed from the spiritual the more people limit their role to that of audience, turning their backs on participation. Dance to be really experienced is something of the body.

Because the layman must use her own, her whole body, in the doing, dance as creative expression presents more problems than participation in the other arts. To-day one is accosted everywhere with GLAMOUR. How can the ordinary "social worker, housewife, factory worker" compete physically with the frothy perfection of the massuered, corseted, magic-brassiered, manufactured composite of a female. The adult who seeks self-expression in dance has a difficult time in believing that her "natural" body is important enough to warrant the time, the money, the effort to learn to use it as an instrument of expression, especially when it is for no one's gratification but her own.

To achieve the dignity of self-expression is a positive affirmation of self-worth. It is not artificial, it cannot be bought, it can exist only through the student. The teacher must help and guide and indeed needs to utilize insight, intuition, experience and original pedagogic methods. Her own objective must be pure: to work toward the utmost development of the individual student. "From the engine shaft to the driving wheels" of the student and from there onward to see "not alone wheels but wings in the air". (E)

There will always be professional art and we shall always look to it as existing for the world and not alone for the artist. There is also room for the humble. There doesn't seem to be, but if the amateur wants it she must try to carve a little space for self.

Artistic creation is a labyrinthine valley of experience. It is also the towering mountain where, despite the distance from the top, one can feel the sun's warmth through walking slowly on the low winding road below.

THE END

REFERENCES

BE: Blanche Evan "I am the Sun" Dance Magazine. March 1950

CS: Curt Sachs. World History of the Dance

E: Ezekiel

F:W   Freud as presented by Waelder

HC: Henry Caudwell: The Creative Unconscious

J: Job

HE: Havelock Ellis: The Dance of Life

Pamela's Dream
A Case History
Fall 1962
by Blanche Evan

This material was originally published
in Packet of Pieces by Blanche Evan,
Private Publication, N.Y.C., 1978

Pamela's Dream

This is an unedited transcript of tape presented to my inner circle of trainees in dance therapy. The long_____means the tape could not be heard clearly. "No notes will be taken and the content will remain confidential."

Pamela we shall call her was a referral from a psychotherapist (whom we shall refer to as Dr. X) in the beginning of her therapy. The client was 20. She had acted, danced and modelled since the age of 4.

The cast of characters:

Pamela, between 20 and 25 years old; a mother who drinks heavily though always holds down a job; grandmother: dead eight years; family women: aunts, cousins, half sisters; father, in absentia for the major part of Pamela's life. She had seen him once when she was three and once when she was seven. He is now dead. Mac Crist an acrobatic teacher; Olcott, short term lover; Dr. X and three other MD's for check ups; and myself, the dance therapist.

In the interview I learned that Pamela had been a child model from the age of 4 years until 12. She was coerced into acrobatic dance and the ballet and theater. She was really a child bread-winner. Always subjected to criticism of her body; always disapproved of her own body. "Prayed to be thin." Much self observation in mirror, both dressed and in the nude. "Looking and wishing for a change in body contour." Grandma had acted and had been thoroughly accomplished in the theater arts. Mother had been an exhibition dancer with one of our famous ballroom studios. In a typical day, when it was to seek a job, she said, "Well, the usual preliminaries: primed and primped for try-out."

In answer to a request to shut her eyes and give me a body image, she included every part of the body, even to the shape of the head, the length of folds, proportions, etc. But made absolutely no mention of arms and hands. When questioned, however, when she was finished describing her body image, she had a great deal to say about them, including: "Upper arm too plump, hands can be graceful but they can also be ugly during housework and drudgery, gray, old, wrinkles like alligator hide."

She described some eczema on her hands during childhood. Mother's physical actions were described with excitement. She said she had, "A perfect Yul Brynner stride." Big-boned, strong, capable hands. Pamela still thought of the theater as an exciting place. Her conception of dance therapy was muscular blocks to response. There was no thought, no feeling of movement as expression. She also indicated that she hates lying on the floor when dancing.

I believe that in this particular case, dance therapy can play a most instructive role for the patient, to replace the social criticisms, the family rejections and self-disapproval of the body, with a body image closer to her own nature and then to help rebuild it accordingly. Pamela approves of her body proportions on the whole. We set to work on what she <u>disapproved</u> of. She disapproved of the proportions of the shoulder span to the rest of the body, and when we worked, she said, "It hurts, but it's a nice pain."

She said that she had no breath endurance <u>except when she was angry</u> and in a mad scene in the theater she could run or perform for minutes and minutes and minutes and never give out of breath. Hands are very symbolic to her. Leaving hands and arms out of the body image I think, of course, is significant. The therapist, when I said this to her on the phone, interpreted this in this way: She said she cannot grasp the realities of her life. But I say, in addition, she is also ashamed of her hands.

I think she's ashamed, as perhaps representative of the burden of taking care of all the housework since the age of 12, because when her grandmother died all the breadwinning stopped and she became the maid in the house; the mother went to work and Pamela stayed home and took care of the house at the age of 12 until the time that she went into therapy and after. Even when we were working on the shoulder, she said, "It feels like I'm walking somewhere, with my hands, that is." They also represent to her, I think, her inability and frustration in her competition with mother, who as the bread-winner and strong, seems to be a man, I think. "She has big bones, "she said, "Whereas mine are little." Pamela's stance is that of an over grown baby doll, wide and inert, and her walk is weightless.

She loved the physical appearance of the studio in this first session. She thought it was very beautiful, and she was fascinated by the drums: she was looking at them. I think that when we get to playing them, this will help in developing a positive hand and arm strength and channel for expression of aggressiveness as well as an outlet for hostility.

My personal response to this client was one of an all out desire to help, along the lines described to her by me, that dance therapy was finding the relation between the problem and the body. From this point, I will not say what is second, third, fourth, fifth session, but I will give you the reports in sequence. "How did you get along this week?" I asked Pamela the next time I saw her. She said, "Very well." She felt much better; she accepted some invitations to go out and the strain in the neck and the head seemed much relieved, and we worked on shoulders. I asked her about the comment she had made the last week when she had mentioned body tension, and I asked her now where this was. She said, a numbness in the legs and the lower arm and a sensation of muscles in the lowest back as if pulling apart horizontally. I said,"When?" She said, especially after reading a long time. I asked her to show me the position in which she reads, and it was obvious that circulation would be stopped in this position because both legs were together and swung under the hips, and the arms pressed on the chair, and yet she had no idea that this, in itself, would cause a blocking off of circulation.

I suggested a different kind of position for the following week: untwist it and I suggested that at times she stretch out. I asked her if there were any other times, she said, yes: pre-menstrual pain. And then she said she felt this tension in repeated nightmares when she awakened in a cold sweat and in the nightmare someone, and always the same person, was in uncontrollable violence to Pamela.

I asked the patient to walk around and if she had any image of herself walking. "None," she said. She said she had never watched herself walk. This was interesting. In contrast to the detailed image of her body in static stance which she had given to me. Then she said she knew a few things about it though. For instance, she said she could not stroll and she could not stand slowness in anyone walking in front of her, and as she said this, she imitated a very sick looking creature. So I got up and walked in front of her very straight, but she said, no, the reaction was the same. She had to get in front and move faster. And she refers frequently, both last week and this, to her ability to wind in and out of crowds and to get ahead fast. She said she couldn't stand the slow walk of the choir, for instance. I asked her to run. She said it was hard to run without imagining a situation, like running after somebody. And in, I think I mentioned this before, in reference to a lack of endurance, she said that she could run for an hour after somebody in a scene.

I must say at this point that I've worked with a number of people in the theater and this should be a chapter in itself: actresses and actors in therapy. And she said again she had indefinite endurance when mad and this I think is very very important to remember. While she was running in her typical weightless way, on two or three steps I heard her feet on the ground, and this led to a very important revelation, because when I brought this to her attention, she said, "Oh, I never put my feet on the floor. I always walk on the toes because it's easier to move." She said, "And I have flat feet, both of them, and they are a hindrance and they are ugly."

I explained what a terrific strain she had been putting on the legs and spine and asked her to stand with her heels on the ground, and she immediately showed me how the whole foot touched the ground, how ugly it was. It took no more than two minutes before I had her foot muscles working so the lifted arch was there and high enough for a pen easily to be slipped under the arch. It was agreed that she would practice this daily even when in her street shoes, and as she was doing the exercise, she pulled her hand into a very predatory position, of tremendous intensity as she was doing the arching_____. (Very young children simultaneously muscularize hand & foot, arms & legs).

Then she became self-conscious and she said that this really should be a foot exercise, she thought, and I said, no. I told her again what dance therapy was, and I think this is very interesting in relation to what creative dance is in relation to what dance therapy is. And I told her that she was certainly <u>free to involve her hands emotionally</u> when practicing her footwork at home. Then I explained how she had been carrying all her weight on the little bones of her feet for some years--that was working them worse if there were any arch problem at all.

I asked her to carry some drums. She found this very easy and I asked her to lie down and put one of our big drums on her diaphragm to see about her breathing capacity and she had absolutely no trouble. She seemed to have tremendous breath capacity even with this big weight on her. Then she demonstrated how flexible her fingers were.

We worked on different kinds of walk the next time, basic kinds, to activate the feet. The explanation of them required a slow tempo for their doing; in order to explain to her how these walks were done, I had to do it slowly and she did it slowly. And when we sat down, she remarked how that was the first time she had ever enjoyed slow walking. In each session she had mentioned her irritation at walking behind a slow person in the street, and her need and her ability to get out of the situation.

I had wanted to pursue this, since tempo is a basic element of movement of dance, and therapy. I asked her if slow movements of any person in any other situation bothered her and this led at once to a description of the movements of her mother, from which one could conclude that Pamela's mother consumed, not only all the space in the house, in a small apartment where the mother throws the clothes all over and absolutely absorbs it all, but she also consumes all the time in the house. And Pamela went into that further, that when they were going to the theater, at the last moment the cosmetic business would go on and Pamela would watch the clock and know that they were going to be late and there was nothing that could hasten this woman to move.

Or when the mother took a bath. She would stay in the tub for ages, and Pamela would say, what can she be washing so long. And this has been going on all of Pamela's life. Now, I think that these points are important because sometimes when we dance a great deal, we are apt to think of tempo always as beat and rhythm and so forth. But tempo is here being used really as part of the whole life picture, not in the sense that we work the tempo in dance particularly, and yet it is a very important part of dance therapy. And I recalled an old definition of mine about dance in which I said: "space, time, body movement dynamics and content welded in unity." And this is the approach that I use always in my work in therapy, too.

Now further discussion led to Pamela's own expression of slowness. I asked her certain questions and so forth. And she said that when she was 13, Pamela had worked out an effective way of losing weight because she was so unhappy with her weight, though I had seen pictures of her and she wasn't really very fat. It's just that she's been told always, that with all this weight she wouldn't get jobs. She'd be rejected for this play; she wouldn't get this modelling job--and this is what had been thrown to her and this is what made her be so unhappy about her weight.

So she had worked out this thing all by herself of not eating and being inactive at the same time, and she did lose a lot of weight. And the mother was very angry at all that at the time. And then in recent years, she said that in the morning she would, after doing all the chores and getting her mother out to work, she would think of all the many things she would do in the house the moment her mother left, and yet the moment she did leave, she would lie down and do nothing. She wouldn't read. She would do nothing. And I pointed out that this part of the slow tempo perhaps was a protest and really a very destructive one to herself. And perhaps her annoyance with the slow tempo of the people in the street might also be a protest, destructive to her feelings about people.

We picked up the matter of the hands in different ways, and one of the ways was this: I suggested that she look at pictures of hands in the arts, and this threat of her feelings about her ugly hands of which I was so aware in the first session and naturally, when she excluded them from the body image. And so I suggested this matter to her. And she in turn mentioned the strength of her hands. She said that she could throw a telephone book and the sound noise of the telephone book, "makes me want to cry."

This is important as you will see when we go on into the next session. I posed two problems for Pamela for this session. One, to assume the physical characteristics in movement of anyone who at anytime had rejected her on the basis of her bodily characteristics, as she had mentioned so often. Or, she would assume the physical characteristics in movement of her mother, as Pamela had described them so often. She had referred to her walk, for instance, and so forth. There was great resistance, but she chose the second one. She chose the mother. She said it was terribly difficult to do this because she didn't want even for a minute to be like her mother. And she had referred to her mother as the huge bulk of her, and so forth. Now, of course, when a patient says things, you don't take them at face value, but you write them down as much as you can.

She began trying by verbalizing things that she had not ever spoken of before, even to have her mother sick on the john--the intimacy in this household was complete. There was absolutely nothing of privacy. And describing other things, but only once in a while as she talked, she assumed the physical posture. And then more happened, and more enactment, and I say what a difference between words and action. For instance, when Pamela in her first session had described her mother's Yul Brynner's stride, and I asked her about that and doing that now, she got up to move but it wasn't a stride at all, it was a very funny looking trot, with an accompanying verbalization of,"Oh, I must get there, oh dear, oh dear," and her left arm swinging and it was really a very ridiculous picture of a big woman walking in the street.

Pamela suddenly became aware of this and I reassured her that whatever she revealed in movement in the studio was as confidential as whatever she revealed in words to her psychotherapist. And this helped. And from that moment on, she became more and more free in enacting physical postures of her mother and then unnoticeably switched from present to the past. I have explained that we were trying to take things out of her mind where they had been brewing and to begin to let them out through the channel of the body. She was talking and crying and enacting in full intensity, and she re-experienced three episodes one after the other in which her mother had exerted actual violence.

Her mother's words, her actions and Pamela's own physical and emotional reactions, all at once. She pressed her hands against her ears--she said to protect them, "My ears always hurt," and to shut out the harsh words. And then she said--she enacted the action of her mother, slapping her full across the face and so strong that it spun her around as she was enacting it, remembering, "Why does she hate me so, and why am I here at all." This is what she remembered from her childhood when this incident had happened.

And then the enactment of her mother throttling her by clutching her coat collar. Now, there are more descriptions of all these incidents, more details, and I just couldn't get them down fast enough because this patient screamed out--only a tape recorder could have done it--words, tears and actions. I can tell you--I was riveted against the wall. I had never seen such a complete enactment with such intensity, with such vividness, and such abandon as this person exhibited. I said not a word. When it was all over, I asked how old she had been the last time her mother had hit her, and she said, "When I was in junior high school--I was 15."

The next time she came, because these sessions were very very long--she said that after her last session with her therapist, she felt straighter--she had no breathlessness and she was enjoying the air and the day, and she felt that she wanted to get up in the morning and she was better in trying on dresses, and she was going about more slowly, but in a different way. She said, "I feel more a whole being." I told her that we were going to concentrate on her evaluation of her own body--who had rejected it and why--her responses, her present ideal and ways of accomplishing it--and that from now on, we must work for a daily changing of body in relation to the realistic ideal we attained.

We reviewed the exercises and I added some. She said that she had been rejected "because I was fat." I asked if she'd ever been called names. "Yes," she said, "butterball face" and "Parrel the Barrel" was a nickname.

She dieted at 6 years for modelling, which started at 4 and until the age of 13. And I gave her more exercises to do. She said the family was very athletic, "swinging and batting each other to hell." Their standard, "meant more to me than myself." And then she became very conscious of the fact that she might go back to the family some day and compete with them, with her athletic cousins. She said, "Now that I feel better, I think I could do that." Well, I stopped her right there and pointed out that again she was using "feeling better" to meet their standards instead of creating her own. And she caught on and she said, yes. Her body was always judged by her and others for its "commercial use." And then she said, "Beauty is to me saleable."

I questioned her and she said she believed this up until six months ago and I said, "Well, why did you stop?" She said because depression took over and nothing was beautiful nor saleable nor anything. I discussed the disparity between her verbal description of her mother's walk--the Yul Brynner stride in her first session with me and that silly little trot she had enacted in the last one. She said, "Mother's walk is divided--the Yul Brynner stride is for show, but the trot is used by her in her personal life."

Pamela feels now that she is too plump in the upper arms and that she knows that some of this she says is hereditary--again, a tie up with the family. I mentioned again her daily doing of things, the coming week, to change her body daily.

The next time when she was supposed to be here, she called instead, and said she'd gone downstairs to make the call and that she was "developing a block to these lessons." And for the last 24 hours she had wanted to call me to cancel but hadn't, and she had a hoarse voice because she was angry at herself, and "Mother's been sick for two days and in bed 24 hours a day and the house is going to be painted in February," and she went on and on and on. And I didn't say very much. I simply said, "Are you well?" She said, yes. I said, "Then you could be here in half an hour." And she was here in half an hour.

Now, she had not seen her psychotherapist for about 10 days, so that when she got here, she began to talk and she talked and talked. And she talked in material which really did not relate to the dance therapy work, except for about 15 minutes of it. However, I let it go on. She seemed desperate in her need to talk. On the other hand, I felt it was wrong and it didn't belong and I knew that I would have to do something to stop for the future.

I explained this to Pamela. And I explained again what dance therapy was. So then we spent another hour, after spending 2 in just her talking this way--we spent another hour really in dance therapy material. I tried to face her resistance to coming and I thought, at the time, we did accomplish a lot. Part of this related to a new exercise I'd given her in which I had had her lying on the floor and this had triggered her memories of Mac Crist, the acrobatic teacher. And she began to reveal dramatic experiences of her acrobatic training (trainer). I suggested also her possible sense of guilt in having enacted her mother's violence to her and in enacting the mother's physical characteristics which had shown up so poorly really and I reassured her as to the confidential relationship between the dance therapist and the patient, and asked her anything that bothered her in working on the hands and she said, yes, because it recalled her mother's hands.

I asked her if she resented my bringing to her attention that it was time to build her own body image and to stop competing with images created for her by her family. She said she had not resented it but she really couldn't accept it yet. She really wants no goal at this time at all. I told her that eventually she would have to make her choice, her own choice, about whether she wanted to continue to be so affected by the family in regard to body--eventually she would have to make her own choice.

As a dance therapist, I could not let her blindly start another cycle of being rejected for a body standard which she couldn't attain. Since her first life span that had been lived with other people's standards had finally led her to depressions and immobility. I pointed out to her that regardless of any feeling or neurotic reasons for breaking appointments, she had social responsibilities to appointments, to me, and that if they were to be cancelled, they were to be done so in time. I think that you all know enough about therapy to understand the importance of these attitudes of mine to the patient's behavior. To say briefly, for instance, that instead of accepting the fact on the phone, that she wouldn't come, that, quite simply, I got her to come, and how important it was for what transpired. And that I saw no reason why she should not be made aware of the fact that she has responsibility, in time, to the therapist. And I know all the other answers and the reasons, too, and the whys, but I am--I feel very strongly about patients developing a sense of social responsibility and--they can still fit in the transference or reasons that come up.

I then sent a note to the therapist: "Pamela's case seems to me one of antipathetic symbiosis (antipathetic being destructive and symbiosis being great dependency), her very body bound up with that of her mother's, and this is true 24 hours a day in the apartment in which they live. This goes into the daily routine as well into the management of the house and in the cooking and the girl's conflict--she doesn't really want to give up these chores because she takes pride in it and it makes her feel superior to her mother, I think, and so forth. Now, although she knows that her mother consumes both the time and the space and that at some point she will also consume Pamela if given a free rein, she is not ready to leave her mother even theoretically, and I certainly never proposed it. But I feel that the more she pulls out the injury from memory, the greater the pull to her mother will be at this time, for many reasons. And I feel that the next period of therapy in my work will be much more difficult than it has been up to now.

Pamela loved the work on the hands until her hands and actions reminded herself of her mother's hands. In other words, when she looked at her own hands, she sees her mother's. She would be perfectly willing to drop the studies in hands and art, as I have suggested; on the other hand, Pamela's hands are a symbol also to herself of inferiority--of her mother's domination--of her house drudgery. She wants to work on beautifying her hands and she can do so only until the moment when they appear to her to be those of her mother's, and then all work is blocked.

Anybody who is given to Pamela as an exercise is traumatic to her, either instantaneously or within a few hours or days and this is a girl who danced for years and years and years. This is why exposing her to the general and unproducable of the group would be destructive to her and I would not permit her to enter a group, and I never did. Nor would she herself consent, though I have never even discussed it with her. To help Pamela best, I think it wise to give her more opportunity at enacting through improvisation and just forget about the exercise at this time, not, however, to rule out exercise, but to help her disassociate from a previous experience. For instance, to use the hand studies, to remake Pamela's hands image, of her hands to herself, so that she can see them as hers and not as those of her mother's, because the whole purpose of mine in studying hands and the world and trying to get her hands identify, was to bring them out into the light, <u>because she had hidden them in that first session</u>.

Pamela, even when she was little, did stand back and contemplate the reasons for her mother's and grandmother's behavior, and I think it was this ability at objectivity which saved her, and, therefore, I felt from the beginning, that this had a very hopeful prognosis, because I felt the girl herself had, all the way up, through all the torture, exhibited a way of asking to herself, why is this happening, why am I treated this way. Pamela, when she said, "beauty is saleable," she said she believed this for 15 1/2 years. I feel that her mother and grandmother prostituted her body from the age of 4 to 12--they were selling her body. How to help her recreate the basic evaluation of her body, to build her own acceptable body image for the sake of self and dignity, how to increase her feeling of safety which was the feeling that the psychotherapist had suggested to me to try and instill in the girl, in her body--how to build her self-confidence--I think is tantamount to breaking the symbiosis on a physical, always the psycho-physical level.

Again, at the time that Pamela was due for the next session, her mother called--this is the first time the mother spoke to me and she went on and on and on and on and couldn't get a word out of me--found me very non-conversant. And then Pamela got on the phone and then finally she arrived a half hour later and her mother called again to see if Pamela had arrived. And it was all explained and in fact, the mother had given her 15 cents for the bus so she wouldn't take a taxi, and very interesting, the girl asked the doorman for money and came in a cab anyway.

I explained to Pamela that I thought she was permitting her mother to make Pamela into her own image, to make her slow up, to make her late, for the theater, and for this and for that and for getting out of the house, and so forth, and this is just what Pamela had so often resented and yet she was letting her mother make her into the same kind of slow getting out from the purpose--and we enacted together my interpretation of this kind of influence, and_____, and she grasped it--I think it got in front of her and it kind of hypnotized her, although I know nothing about hypnosis. But I just walked in front of her, like this, and she just walked backwards and we walked like that and like that and she knew, much better than I could say in words, what I meant by this insidious kind of influence that the mother was wielding over her.

Pamela spoke of the horrible three nights in a real nightmare she had had, which was a little bit of what you saw--and she had awakened this morning with a terrible pain in the back of her neck, and the arms out and the hands clamped in a kind of rigor mortis, with her left hand lifeless and paralyzed. From this point on, just as in the enactment of her mother's violence, she talked so fast and so much, that it was impossible to take it down, but this was the best I could do, and everything I write now is a quote:

"A group of women, a whole family of women want something out of me; they are after me. Somebody is doing something with their arms. Heavy legs all of them, coming toward me, going to do something to me, who is where, who is where, brunettes and gray hair and woke up with the name of my cousin on my lips and my mother's first cousin and there was a white house with a black and a family gathering and everybody's going to get into one big fight in a room and I'm very small.

There are two couches and a big lamp and a chair and I'm trying to hide but mother or grandmother says, 'do come here and talk to so and so--do, dear, come here and do this and this and the other--and do come come and do this and that'--(in deep commanding voices which I cannot imitate)--and then an uncle and aunt and the house disappears--and people are standing--and it's cold, terribly cold--and I have to go to the toilet. And their mouths are moving and their voices are not individual--all from the person but more as if the sky were talking--and then enough, and as small as I could get and I want to be underneath the ground." (And, of course, she was talking and crying at the same time, but she hadn't done anything with her body--she was just_____.)

I had tried to get Pamela to enact her nightmare but she was in a terrible agitated state and I felt that I must pull her back to the physical reliving in her body--of the nightmare. So I became very firm and said, "Stop talking and move," which she did, and very soon after, while she was dancing out the nightmare, she broke into free tears which didn't happen when she was talking, and she went on moving and talking and crying.

At this point, when she was wanting to be under the ground, tied in a knot, I pulled that blanket out, which is magic in the studio--it's worked in a thousand different ways--and I threw it to her and she buried the upper part of her body under it and around it, lying on the floor that way. Then she went on talking: "For oblivion, nothingness, gray, no feeling, lightness, touching yourself and you are yourself or have other people bother me--I don't want to touch myself with my hands and have the entire--hands must feel my body like a corpse--I'd be plaster--smoke--heavy as in the texture of smoke."

When she was finished I asked her to look at her hands. She said, "Reddishwhite knuckles--they're dry and red--and I see two spots on them and there are five fingers and a palm." And I asked her about the color of her nail polish. Don't ask me why. I don't know why I asked her that. She said, "Frosty pink." And I said, "Your mother's?" "Dried blood red," she said. An then with a horrible cynical gesture she added, "Victory red." I asked her to press her hands on her face and touch it. She said, "face is cold, mealy-like, like cold oatmeal. It's really hot now and flushed but my hands are an entity--my skin is grainy--textured wall paper - in the dream I still want to touch my body--I haven't liked it for so long."

I asked when she could remember the first time she didn't like her body and she said, "When I had my first cold and I was all stuffed up and I couldn't cry or talk or drink water or breathe, and there were bars on the crib." I said, "How old?" "Two years old," she thought. I said, "were there clamps on the crib blanket--the words that you used to describe your arms when you woke up out of your nightmare." She said, "yes, yes, yes--that seems right." And she went on about a tall doctor being there and so forth. "Yes," she said, "the clamps--it doesn't seem right--and I was always tucked in with the clamps." I think you remember that, when she wakes up, with her hands like clamps. "I was always tucked in and until 7 1/2 I sucked the second and third fingers of my right hand, sucking and hiding under the blanket, while the other hand pulled little bits from the blanket.

I asked Pamela again to look at her hands and to try to see hers instead of her mothers. And she said, "They were nine_____--when I was about six and a half or so, I was more feminine then--like my last year in high school. I don't know where that went, I don`t understand what masculine is--not feminine, nor masculine--I feel like an oddity."

Then Pamela said to me, "You asked me to see myself through my mother's eyes and I tried it, and I came to the bosom sticking out like a shelf, her bosom is so big she can't see anything beyond it, and all the women in the family are that way." She said, "Mine are so small." She said, "They're all masculine women--like the prow heads the ships, sort of sailing. Grandmother's walk," and she began to move again, --Stomp--stomp--stomp--very strong steps with a side to side movement of her shoulders--up and down, too, as a man might have. She said, "Grandma could look like a man walking beside me or with me--her face is that of a man." And she spoke about picking at her body after grandma died. And I said, "Did it hurt?" And she said, "Yes, at times." She said, "It was like trying to get something out of my body."

She said before 10 she had had a mole. She said that grandma had lots of them, thousands of them--"I had only some." So I said, "Were you pleased that you had only some or would you have rather had lots like grandma?" She said, "That's fantastic your saying that. Because just yesterday I was looking at this big spot (which is part of a skin illness that she had) and I thought how that was the exact place on the inside of my right ankle where grandmother had had it also."

Just as grandma," she said.

"My voice and quality and sometimes the same as in mother's words. Then I want to kick her"-- and she's talking about her mother then, and Pamela gave her leg a free swinging, hard kick, she said, "So she'd land on her face. I want to kick her right between where it hurts"--which, of course, is a very masculine image--because it's like hitting the scrotum--and she too, was really thinking of her mother as a man. She said, "A year and a half ago I slapped her because I'd come in the door and something in her face - and she said, "dear, dear--" and I said, "Had you slapped her at any other time?" And she said, "yes, when she was lying there in her lover's apartment, drunk like a big bloated baby." I said, "A girl or a boy baby?" She said, "A girl. Mother could be very feminine when she dressed to go out and with beautiful clothes and feminine and that I wanted to possess her, to be with me, and not for her to go out and look that way for somebody else."

When I had gone into the dressing room to call Pamela for the beginning of her session, I found her doing an exercise on the floor, and I explained to her that today her full time had been spent really in dance therapy to her advantage. She said, "Yes. Last week--" and this is a great thing that happened - she said last week she had been very disappointed after the session because there had been no physical action. I'm so glad that I pulled her verbalizing today into action--really making her move when she would have not moved without really being pushed into it.

I explained to Pamela what all the material seemed to confirm, that her body was so much part of her mother and grandmothers, that our task was to find her own body again, and to go on from there. And she said she had to leave home and I said, well, that might be so, but it was no use just using that as a delay mechanism, for the problem that faced us in finding the self identity. She then recalled how, when she practiced the piano when she was a little girl, her left hand--you remember the left hand?--couldn't manage the bass and grandmother had sat there always with a stick and rapped her knuckles with it____ ____. I said, "The same hand that was paralyzed this morning when you woke up after the nightmare?" She said, yes, the same. I asked Pamela to try very hard that if the nightmare happened again, because she said that when she awakes, she throws the cover off and she goes to the toilet. I said to try and use her arms and hit out with them. She has said that in her dreams she can never move to defend herself--(END OF SIDE 1, TAPE 1--SIDE 2 FOLLOWS)

--and I asked her to try to dream moving in the dream and when I discussed my suggestions with the psychotherapist, she approved of the suggestions--I suggested them first and discussed them later--but I did really always want to check with her.

Pamela, the next time, said that yesterday, for the first time, she had looked out of the window, participating with the scene, and she felt she was beginning to deal with things--these are her words: "deal with--contend with--and adjust"--and that she was closer to stop rationalizing and replacing this by feeling. I did not question her about this. She mentioned how many devices she had resorted to in her life, "How not to cry." And she spoke of to be not away from home, but "out of it." That she had belonged to "two women and manipulated by them, like on a string." I brought up the use of the words in the last session of duality and plurality. Pamela said she was referring to the action of our session in the sense of duality because she felt so tense--she was building a block to coming here and yet she wanted to, and that's the sense of duality with her, and she doesn't know why--when I said "and plurality"--and she said, "Oh, that's an embellishment,"--and that's what I mean about people attached to the theater--the watching out for the thing that creeps in--that is really theatrical and which is perfectly valid because that's been a major part of their life and I'm sure if a dancer were in movement therapy, there would be a great deal there that one would have to realize came out of dance and perhaps was a layer above the therapeutic situation.

But most of all I wanted to explore her reference to herself as an oddity. And she said, "Mother had explained when I was nine or ten, that men are the stronger sex, and that men always disappointed mother because they never lived up to their promise--not their potential, but their promise. And also, that all the marriages had been unhappy ones--grandmother's, mother's, and aunts, and so forth. "Sex--a disturbing role." "Being an oddity--where do you start from--feeling neuter is a shield that is always there." She said there was safety in it--something to hold onto. "So when I see girls tittering"--and by that I think she meant coy or feminine--she said, "I resent it because if I tried to act feminine, I might not know how to." And this is the world who for all the world looks like a budding women - there is nothing masculine in this girl's appearance at all.

Now we hadn't referred to Olcott before but this was a short term love affair that she had had--that meant a lot to her. I said that, "Olcott brought out your femininity." She said, yes, and she enjoyed it. And I tried to refer to the "massive, big bosomed women" that she'd always mentioned--and she said, "I can't understand men. These masculine women, like mother and grandmother, say they are capable of doing anything a man can do--they pick out weakness in men and exaggerate them because they feel inadequate as women." (She had analyzed all this--this was pretty wonderful.)

"Even grandmother, who had three older brothers, and was daddy's little girl, competed, so that eventually she could outrun her brothers and and this frustrated them."

Of course, these were very castrating women, and, either she was too weak, in the sense that she felt too inadequate to cope with them, maybe that saved her--or, she was very strong, she was very strong--and I really think it was the strength--from everything that I know about her. In every case, she really didn't want to accept the standard for herself of a masculine women. She said, "The women's masculinity--all my senses were touched by them--hearing the loud, deep voices--seeing their walk and feeling grandmother's hand on my shoulder or on my back--and mother's hand on my face when I was slapped - and grandma pushing me. I had to be important. I wanted to be something. I had to be. But I was born second best because I was a girl."

I said to her, "Femininity to you is a big risk. Yet you enjoyed your feminine role with Olcott and your femininity in your last year at high school, as you had mentioned." She said, yes, and she clings to this short love experience that she had had. Then I asked her--I said I would ask a few questions and to please answer the very first thing that came into her head. I said, "What is the worst thing that ever happened to you?" And she said immediately and self-consciously, "Well, my mind is blank. I don't know what happened. There are two or three people in a light, new dress and I am extremely small and they are very big."

And from this point on I will refer to the nightmare very often, though I didn't refer to it when I spoke to Pamela, because in the nightmare, of course, she is extremely small - that is the thing that is so terrifying to her and find that she winds herself up in a knot and gets under the ground. And I asked, "Now that you think out the question, what is the worst thing that ever happened to you, instead of an immediate response, what is your answer?" She said--and again it was the incident of her mother: "My mother washing the clothes and she slapped me across the face when I was nine. I couldn't move. But I had to move to get out of her violence and I was terrified. I couldn't move." That, too, was in her nightmare--"I couldn't move."

I said, "What is the thing you want most in the world?" And she said, "Round, Something round and nebulous and soft." And I said, "If you think it out?" And she said, "Well, I want a father and a country and a big house." Now, that was in the nightmare, too - but I wanted well. She said, "Life is hell. It's a lot of bull and a disappointment."

I said, "Can you formulate what you would like your therapy to lead to?" "And to work out." This is her answer: "The confusion about myself. What to do. I want to be something in between--neuter, it, sexless. It's strange and peculiar--neither boy nor girl. I didn't know until the second or third grade that I was a boy or a girl. Because from 3 years old into kindergarten and for years thereafter, grandmother dressed me in many clothes - clothes - under corduroy pants I was boxed in--what was she keeping away--other little girls were dressed in cute frills above their knees and Mary Janes - how I wanted frills and Mary Janes--even the household was strange, living in one room." She named the girl friends that she's had in the seventh and eighth grades, searching to find out why they were feminine. I asked her how long she had had this break out on her skin and she told me a long time. and I said,"You'd mentioned something on your arms____ ____ ____". and it seems that at various times her skin had reacted to her emotional problems.

Then she said, in the 4th and 5th grades, for 2 1/2 years, she had had a fungus between the thumb and the first finger on the writing hand and then she explained that her grandmother had forced her to practice the Palmer system of penmanship every day for hours.

I had determined that no patient would leave a session without working physically. I told Pamela I had prepared a few moving projects and if the first one was not good for her to do today, that I would suggest the others, but she wanted the first. It was based on part of her last week's when enacting "being little" she had, after a moment on the haunches, stood up to enacting little, and I had insisted that she enact it really crouched down, making herself as little as possible.

She said it's harder to be little. So I went back to this and I drew the analogy for her____ _____that it really was harder for her to be her age and little, just as it was physically with her body to really be little. The moving_____was to be little, to do really a_____--she at once made herself tiny; then she said, oh, you wanted it down, so I said, no, never mind. She was sitting hunched over on the floor with her legs up to her chest--"and six inches across the back, an inch long here, four inches high, my head is down, I remember being that small, I had been bathed and was standing on the john, and both parts were down and I was standing being dried and I slipped and fell down between the wall and the john - I was so scared I couldn't cry."

And remember in the nightmare, and in another carriage____ ____that she always had, she couldn't ever talk or cry in addition to not being able to move. "I had tried to say something and couldn't," and as she enacted this, she was really trying to make the effort to make a sound--it was all so real to her. "And my chest was so constricted--I couldn't breathe, and grandmother and mother standing there, hysterically laughing."

I asked her if any comfort of any kind of help had been forthcoming--again, because you don't accept this kind of complete rejection. And she said yes--she said she remembered a look of concern on her mother's face and she imitated it. Then she went on, "I spread my legs for room, because I was only two or three or four years old, and they picked me up, and instead of crying, I urinated." You know, at the end of her nightmare, she'd always run to the toilet. She said, "I don't remember if they laughed at that or when I was on the floor. I was small and squished, and later on in school at a desk, I felt small and squished this way, and I hurt the lower part of my back in the fall." You remember that that's where she gets tension. "And my feet were cold and wet, and I had a terrible fear." And then she said,--"I must have been that small, otherwise how could I get down there between the wall and the john?"

Of course, the intensity was now broken--this was an extremely intense experience, really, on the level of intensity, as the others. So she said, "How could I get down there," unless she was small, and then she turned around to herself and she said, "Now, Pamela, don't try to get down behind the toilet."

Which is very interesting because it showed certainly a self-destructive tendency, even though she was aware of this, and she had had suicidal thoughts at times in her life.

And again it showed this characteristic that I found so wonderful of her, of being able to look at something and see it and here it was again. And then she went on, "It is fantastic how small I can be. I'm in a play pen in the Adirondacks, trying to stand on my head, and I saw blue spots and bitter nausea and poison coming into my mouth and through my nose, making myself sick." Again, this self-destruction--"looking through the bars of the play pen and my cousin laughing at me, and then in my crib making funny faces at my cousin and he laughing--already they were laughing at me." And this is very important because she really felt that the world of adults that she knew had only contempt for her. I put on some music then. I think this was the first time that I'd ever put some music on. She said, "It reminds me of a rocker we had, that looked like a witch--it had become alive and I'd hide--the cat(?) coming at me from each corner."--as in the nightmare again.

She had actually had this rocker and she was so terrified of it--it had taken on the appearance of a witch at night and the things were coming at her from each corner, just as in the nightmare. Something alive in the closet and moving, closing in on all sides--and other dreams of insects and so forth. She said, "I wanted to scream but I couldn't." Again that terrible frustration. And when she said this, her right hand fisted: "I wanted to scream but I couldn't." And it really seemed like a real frustration at not being able to attack.

I tried to separate what was experienced and what was the night dream and what was fantasy. She said, "No, the fantasies were day dreams and they have always been pleasant things." So--we had actually not gone into them and actually during the course of the therapy we never did--they were very much relating to her ideal body, you know, thin body, and so forth. And as most children in our society--it's all television--but, of course, in her case, you see, she lived in this house with these two women, and all this terror going on in the television, and then she said, "Actually, once a month I at least murdered one person." And then she would watch some more. And she--the whole place became filled with terror. By the way, which she got over with only after the grandmother died and she threw out very much in the house and redecorated it--she was still a young child.

Now I must tell you at this point that she felt many sweet things about her grandmother, too. I think that she never felt anything sweet about her mother, as far as I can see. But with her grandmother--she felt that there was a great deal about her grandmother that wasn't, despite all these other things--and then she related a recurring_____dream, and so forth here. In one dream, "I was a huge human being," and, of course, this is marvelous. I had told Pamela that if I could put into one word the crux of her dance therapy, it was "separation"--the physical separation of her body from the body of her mother and grandmother.

I twisted my fingers with both hands and said, "When one does this, often one cannot tell which is her own left--there are fingers_____, you know, you get mixed up, you don't know which is your finger after a while. I tore the hands apart and demonstrated how, of course, each hand then was smaller than the entwined hand, and that was where we had to start. With her acknowledgement of the entwinement and the physical breaking of the umbilical cord at the age of 20 and a starting out, not little and stifled, but little, her self growing, her own body, and stance, and so forth.

I elaborated on this and she grasped the whole thing. "That I can say about my body--'it's mine'--I never before thought about it in those words. When I say it, I can hear my voice--it's me. At other times my body doesn't feel, and I don't hear myself when I talk." When she described how little she had felt, she said, "My arms are not long enough to reach--and my legs can't run fast enough--and I'm very little around my neck."

This attitude of mind to her littleness is very important, I think, very very important in the course of her therapy, because I had no desire just to make her feel that--well, she was a big girl--no, to herself she really was very little--but to recognize that this little thing which came from the separation, has the potential of now growing up into a person of her own size. I mentioned again her identity of parts of her body with her mother's, as in the hands. "Yes, my palm looks like an infant's. And in our sessions, when I looked at some of these art hands, I was reminded of my mother's hands--her palm is soft and fleshy and white blood-celled that can envelope and eventually absorb_____and_____whisk it away." I say she is alerted of being careful of being consumed by her mother and I reinforced this idea in some discussions.

I also went into details about her body standards, identified in her thinking that her family's psychologically in terms of her heredity and all of that, and the necessity to break this conceptual tie. Well, you know, these sessions are very long, and one would think, well, that was enough, but it wasn't enough for her. She began to move around the room, walking. She said, "Do you notice anything different in my walk?" I said, "It seems natural." She said, "Yes--my feet." And she pointed to them and displayed a very good arch, and she remembered about her flat foot theory, which she had talked about in the first session.

She said,"And my hips are moving when I walk, as a woman's does." She said, "I never walked that way before." And she went to the bar and she did a plie, and she exclaimed, "I'm alive--my hips are no longer granite, as I felt them to be in every dancing lesson I ever had." And you remember in the nightmare she talked of her body being plastic. She said, "I can back bend, and the hurt in the lower back and the fear is gone. I could never do back bends. The lower back isn't destroying the connection between the hips and the upper back. I never had any feeling in the back. Who hammered it in?" She said, "And I'm little and little and little and my arms don't have to be longer than they are to function."

I was reminded of my impression in the first session of her stance as that of an inanimate doll, and now, for the first time, I found a connection with the plaster and the granite that I didn't know about at that time. And this is very interesting because as a dance therapist your sight, again, non-verbally - what do you see and what does it mean to you and how do you utilize it and how a long time after something that you see becomes explained, and becomes valid, and your sight was right, even though you didn't know the reasons for it.

And this matter of her body being plaster or inanimate or doll like was very very important. Now the change into a human being moving about, and it was so startling, that to help believe it, I remembered cases of hysteria and the recall of the disappearance of the physical defect--it was almost as much of a change as that. Pamela felt tiny--she s_____putting her_____, and tiny and tiny--I feel so tiny. But it was Pamela tiny, free--and free to move and to grow and grow up and a_____of Pamela, tiny, tied in a knot, as she had said, and "stifled and unable to talk, tried to scream," and so forth, as she had experienced both in life and in her nightmare. She spoke of the inner confidence since her last session, when she was with her mother, and that she loses this confidence when she's alone, and I spoke of the necessity for changing-

-changing the style of life--which is an Adlerian term which is very good and useful--in small daily patterns. For instance, she had developed the habit of never being dressed in the house, but always being in a robe, and when she had spoken of not being able to stand any more of anything, the nagging of her mother--I said, simply: "Well, why don't you go out--go for a walk?"

She said, "Well, I can't. I'm not dressed." And this change--a simple change in her style of life in the household was very important, because what happened was that she began to be dressed all the time, which, in itself, was a very good thing. It gave her much more of a sense of dignity and she felt always ready to take herself out of this situation, and the result was a lot of the nagging stopped, because her new independence and her new appearance and attitude, of course reacted upon her mother.

Before she left that session, her sinuses began to flow out free one Kleenex after another. And I recalled her enacting her scenes in the pen when she was standing on her head and the poison for what_____to herself, and she was making herself sick in her own words, and so forth, and I felt this might have been a very definite tie up to that which had occurred.

The next session. Pamela seemed a new Pamela today. She was relaxed and enthusiastic. There was a skin--still continued to break out at times, and she walked in with a big shopping bag of pictures and showed me all the pictures of her whole family, and it was very interesting because I was sure that I had met her grandmother--I knew exactly--she looked exactly the way I had imagined her. And now I will tell you something which is even more interesting than that.

Pamela had associated me with her grandmother, and I didn't know this until after the therapy had ceased, and she had lost it only a month and a half before we terminated the therapy. And we had a discussion about it and she said, "Well, it was mostly because it was my grandmother who was with the dancing all the time," and all of that. And some of this was hard for her to take. And I asked her was there anything pleasant and then it was she told me that she felt sweet things about her grandmother, too. It must have been, because otherwise she could not have given so much in the therapy session.

Now her mother, too, looked as if I had seen her somewhere, but not so much as the grandmother. And the father looked young--had a <u>dreamy look</u>. And Pamela said that he might have been a dreamer but he was always selling something and this had influenced her too, in this idea of beauty being saleable because she knew that her father was always selling things.

Now, the picture of herself in childhood, just broke me up because she had the most beautiful eyes and the most beautiful round body--not fat and tubby at all--but just beautiful--with a real light in them--and then you see her being dressed in all these ghastly show costumes, you know, and her whole story really was most piteous. She went "down" with this "little" thing and wanted to do something.

And then she explained that she had had the experience that something had frightened her very much when she was young and it was supposed to be related to her mother. You never know when you use a word what happens and I was lucky it didn't stifle her completely--that she was able to pick up just a little part and do that enactment of falling behind the john.

So she said that when she got back to the apartment that day, that she had felt little, "but," she said, "everything in the apartment looked smaller. She said before that she had felt bigger, but everything in the apartment was bigger than she. She said, too, that the space in the apartment had changed--it had more air in it now. The mother had changed certain of her habits, of possession, and, she said, "There is no mustiness in the air," and that is purely psychological.

I asked how long this "little" feeling had lasted and she said three or four days. "It's more natural now to be little, feeling young--I'm not 45." She spoke of her dreams--the nightmares ceased.

She said the dreams were now, "My size--with my friends--no family--Olcott was in some of them. And then she made one reference to a tight collar on--she didn't associate this with the things she had enacted of her mother trying to choke her. Now this was interesting. She said that when her mother had stepped near her to wake her up, because Pamela also had certain dependencies upon the mother like that, to wake her up, you know--I mean, there was a terrific interchange of dependency there.

The mother had stepped accidentally on Pamela's glasses and Pamela had warned her that if she ever did that again, and did this as she said it--"You'll get the biggest kick you ever had in your life." She said, "Mother went over neatly and sat down in a chair and looked frightened." I asked Pamela if she had retained the softness of body motion since the last session. She said, yes. And I suggested dancing to music for the very first time and she showed me--and she danced with a wonderful limberness and she did very difficult floor acrobatics without any sense of strain emotionally or physically. And they looked beautiful--they didn't have the ugliness of poor acrobatic dancing. She did back bends and balances and she was just lovely to watch.

In relation to back bends, I would like to tell you that this came out, not here, but in her therapy sessions with her psychotherapist--then I had given her that exercise on the floor and she had hated it so, and her head had hurt, and so forth. She went back to the therapist with all this and by then the therapist knew what had transpired because of the constant interchange of thought between us, and she said it had touched off these traumatic acrobatic lessons, and that particular thing which had tortured her, actually her--this man had pulled her in certain ways so that it physically hurt--and her grandmother loved watching this--and she would come home and say to Pamela, "Pamela, do Mac Crist now, do Mac Crist--and it was that thing, of this torturous exercise, and again I say, when you're working in movement, in therapy, you never know--that was something I gave her because of something in her back, and it was wonderful that I gave it to her, and it was wonderful that it was brought forth, because actually, what the therapist explained to her, was that the grandmother was using these acrobatic sessions as a very vicarious sexual experience for herself, and the therapist thought behind this voyeuristic attitude on the grandmother's part, this position that the girl had to get into--the spread legs--and the other part of the man on her--.

Now I'll go on to a little time later, not too much time--a little time later. And this is what I have to say about Pamela: "Pamela is no longer neuter. She is feminine. She has separated her body from her mother's and her family's. Her body is now a different shape from what it had been before. Pamela's hands now exist to herself. They are now graceful, expressive and functionally stronger. Pamela's concept of her littleness has changed to one of height.

And this was brought out in a very interesting way which I will read you a little later. Pamela's night dreams and nightmares have changed to feminine sexual ones. Pamela is aware of each of these changes, and in most cases the initiative to verbalize and to demonstrate them. On the negative side, certain movements that I give her, that are given to any normal group in a body movement class, still are traumatic for her, and she becomes disturbed and usually associates at once with the origins of the disturbance of within the next two or three days. And something happened at that time but we would pick up these things and we would really--they were washed away pretty rapidly. She would work on them herself and try to find out why they touched off certain things.

Now, I would say that if sessions had been of a regular time,--some therapists now a half hour on the clock--that this would have taken about thirty weeks. Because the sessions were several hours long, it was condensed into about three months, which is such a short time, and with her therapist, too. There was a wonderful force in this girl, a bravery and desire for self-preservation, she could not go on living as she had.

The constant interchange of thought between me and the psychotherapist was a great factor in what we were working toward...at my end of it interpretation of mother dependency, and inter-dependency was crucial--as being a physical symbiosis, really, to the extent of body being body. I remember once asking her--she always combed her mother's hair every morning--the mother had long hair--I remembered asking her what she felt when she combed her mother's hair. There was no moment in that house where those two bodies weren't one, and my feeling that the physical thing needed to be broken, I felt that that was the most important contribution that I had to make to this therapy. Also my use of the basic element of stance. And I felt this kind of case was absolutely right with the approaches I was using because of the physical identity there.

This is another session now. She said one set of fears was finished and a new set of fears comes on. But she sees all this, and that's very good. It's much better than just a feeling of euphoria, that now everything is fine. She said that she had seen a wonderful mime on television and she had re-enacted in front of the mirror. She said he had strong arms, but they were different from mother's. And then she said she plays a favorite game: "Let's make myself tiny. Everything else becomes tiny, but I am not tiny, ____ ____ ____being tiny doesn't work anymore. At this moment I'm too tall."

And this is when she used--unconsciously--she didn't know she did it--but I told her later that she had--when she said that she's too tall, she unconsciously put her hand here, like a shelf across the bosom, which was the same gesture she had used when talking about these big bosoms of the women that had so crushed her in their bigness, and now she was doing that unconsciously. Which, of course, means still the identity, but that, too is realistic. And, at least, she feels that her little bosom, even though they're little, really are as big in significance, because--_____bigger, because she feels a woman, and they, with all their bosoms were really men--like men. She said that it doesn't work anymore being tiny because she's too tall and that things at home were smaller and it's more airy and mother drinks less. And she said--she spoke again about granite and death and how she had felt so old always--now this was interesting. And when--the time some years ago, when her mother had offered to give her sleeping pills and they had had a kind of a suicide pact - you know, I'll make you more comfortable and you'll make me more comfortable, and so forth.

"But now when mother is ill, I tell her, 'You're not going to die." and mother answers, 'Nor are you.'" And this thing has meant a great deal to her, this matter of being so small when you break a round thing in two, and she realizes that her mother, too, has changed. She said, "Until 15, mother said we were just like sisters." And what worked out was that the mother wanted to be the older sister to the daughter.

This was so--there were so many confusions and so much neurosis in this setup that it would take lots longer than this one session or lots more than I could explain or the psychotherapist to explain. She said (Pamela): mirror image is no longer "one fantasy talking to another fantasy. I look different, thinner, though I've gained some weight, and taller." She spoke about hands and that the cousin had often pointed out that in their family they all had the same kind of hand and they couldn't cup the hand. She said spaces remain between the fingers and the cousin kept telling this to her all the time--they couldn't use the hand the way children do who drink water out of the hand.

And then she said, "My palm can hold water now." She used her hands very beautifully in an improvisation to some music and she got dizzy in turning and she has no nightmares and she doesn't know quite what she dreams but she feels they are about Olcott, her lover. She had mentioned at the beginning of this session (I had not known anything about this, until just before this session), in the session with the psychotherapist, that the mother, for a number of years, had been giving her stimulants and sedatives by injection when Pamela asked for it. The mother had even intimated a suicide pact should that seem in order.

Now the mother was very wary of the whole thing because she knew that there were people around who were helping Pamela and who were doctors and therapists and she became very cautious and she'd say, well, now, what is Dr. X going to think about that - you know, and so forth and so on. But Pamela still asked for the injections on occasions. And this came out when I discussed with the therapist the matter of her dizziness and she said that until it is established that this girl had no more stimulants and no more sedatives, she will not be able to know whether her dizziness is there or not, to whether it's a result of the drugs. Now these are harmless drugs, as such, but the dependency upon them of course was terrible and the fact that they do make the body toxic if taken too much--and she feels that until Pamela is really finished with all of this, certain things that have been brought out in sessions about which I did not speak tonight, will not be able to be evaluated. Because some of this may come out of fantasies built in when in a certain state of fantasy.

And I think it's wonderful that the therapist was so aware of the physical interchanges with the body that way. Pamela revealed to me that she cannot bear loud noise. Now you noticed that we never used the drums even once. But that--I didn't know that she felt this about the loud noises. The first time I knew it was when she did this to her ears to shut out the mother's and grandmother's voices. But she felt about the drums that they were, when they were played loudly, that it was like people in a frenzy and yelling and it made her very nervous.

And so probably she's one of the few patients who never played a drum in our therapy. In the course of the last session she had said: "I feel every part of my body more than I used to. I want to work with my body. I never had it before. I walk and I exercise because I feel good. My shoulders are much more relaxed. I have arms and hands. I watch my hands, and they are rather pretty."

This is a summary. Characteristics of the dance therapy sessions: The use of enactment in silence rather than improvisations; no use of drums and almost none of music. I used acute sight, picking up indications of body movement or body appearance for the psychological significance. I coupled this with fearlessness in taking risks for the choice of the enactment, even though the material was so traumatic to the patient.

I did permit what seemed at times excessive verbalizations for a dance therapy session, but reached a point, when I made it a rule that no session be concluded without having used physical expression or physical movement even if this were outweighed in time by verbalization. No patient would leave this room without relating with the body. I used tempo and area to help me interpret the material rendered by the patient. and I used such concepts as life style changes, even though these would be changes that would seem to relate to symptomatic changes rather than to growth changes. I used dance of other cultures or arts of other cultures to aid in one important area, that of her hands.

I did not accept the patient's impressions of her own body image as reality--very important. For instance, her flat feet, Until my objective had been achieved I set no limits on the time of the session, even when they ran to three hours and longer. No extra fee was charged for the extra time. My objectives in the case: primarily to help Pamela create self-identity in her body. Secondarily, to help Pamela rebuild her body image as an independent body. Thirdly, to help her change her standards (her beauty was saleable) to beauty as "myself", beauty as potential for the natural satisfactions of life. Fourthly, to help Pamela change her feeling from being neuter and an oddity to being a self-accepting female.

Some of these changes were root changes. Some of them were symptomatic changes. Some of them were life style changes.

--For instance, while Pamela is enacting the mother's violence, did that change Pamela basically. My answer is no because this is not the root. It was rather a manifestation of the root in action--the root was the rejection by the mother which first occurred when she had become pregnant and had not wanted the child at all.

Now, I think that the enactment of these nightmares and the john came closer to root enactment and possibly to very basic--led to very basic changes. I don't underestimate the value of those enactments. I would be very foolish to do so because when I asked Pamela, at the end of everything, what had been the most important session to her, it was that--she had no trouble in finding the answer. Nor do I wish to underestimate the value of symptomatic change in the person's life and in relation to that--something that I didn't bring--it was a letter that I received after dance therapy and who felt that this was tremendously valuable to the patient, even though it was not on the deepest step level.

In other words, how she lived--how she ordered her life from day to day. In passing, I would say that the violence of the mother through the years, in the end helped Pamela far more than an inactive hostility on the mother's part, or an over-charged deceptive sweetness or over-protection might have done. Because at least when the time came, Pamela had something to hit out at, and I feel this very strongly. And that's why I think that was so important to her. She really could put away this thing, you know.

This wasn't anything she thought or felt or this or that--this was something that had happened to her and she could respond to it. And then when the time came, she could think of hitting back at her. Now let's go back to the first session with the hands and the body image, and the fact that I felt it was very significant that she hid the hand and the arm from relating her body image--she didn't physically hide it--it was there--they were both there all the time--but she just left it out of the body image. And don't you remember what the psychotherapist said--that she could not grasp the realities of life and that's why she did not bring the hand to action. And I said that may be so but she felt so ashamed of it in some way. It was only after the hand had been restored to function, that is, when she could cup water with her hand, and to a self sense of beauty in the hand.

I realized that Pamela had hidden the hand from her body image in the first session, because that had been the agent the mother had used to hasten the end of grandmother.

And then I remembered in the first session, too, that she referred to her hand as gray, old, wrinkled like alligator hide--she had said that in the first session--and I think that was the association--to her grandmother. It's very simple. The grandmother was dying and was unconscious for a long time and Pamela was asked by mother to increase the medication. The child was 12. The mother had gone to bed. It didn't happen the first night, so it was tried again the second night.

This would indicate that the dance therapist can pick up details that show themselves and go on from there toward health without necessarily knowing even the basic traumatic experience. And it is reasonable to believe that Pamela, who was now made aware of finding--of her forgetting her hand in the body image, that this triggered her revealing this burden she was carrying, to her psychotherapist--she never revealed it to me and she never knew that I eventually knew about it. Do you follow this?

When I did find out about it, which was about half way through therapy, it did not change the treatment of the hand in my administering the dance therapy in any way at all. Skeptics in the therapeutic field might say, well, it might have happened this way and it happened here in physical action and before it came out to psychotherapist. And I say it is what happened that counts.

The enactment of recall, or a better way to say it, recall an action--they were also enactments of physical characteristics of those people who had rejected Pamela and of her mother who had exploited her and of her grandmother who had exploited her also. I think that Pamela's case proved something that a great psychiatrist once said and it was this: "All the life experiences, the inner life history, takes part in the elaboration of the body image. Now, inner life history is also the history of our relation to our fellow human beings and the community in its broadest sense."

Now, a sequence of the dance therapy session in a few words: The hands and the stance--baby doll stance. The feet - the tempo and the space of the house. The enactment of the mother's violence and the mother's walks--the stride and the silly walk. "Beauty is to me saleable"__and then I learned of the euthanasia--though Pamela does not know that I know this. "Do Mac Crist - quote from the grandmother. My feeling that this was an antipathetic symbiosis, the littleness in nightmare and the oddity, the enactment of the john scene, the hermaphroditism of the female, which I brought out to Pamela, and which she brought out to me, and her change to a feminine walk, which we never worked on--we never did a thing about that--that girl walked into the studio and at the end of that session she began to walk around and asked how she appeared.

Then her dancing to show music and feeling happy about it. And my learning of the injections given by the mother of stimulants and sedatives. Parturition achieved. And then water washes away sin - the hand is restored to function. As to timing, in pace, she said. "I have no time to stroll out to be aware of slow people"--she was much too interested and busy living and being Pamela. Then I say, the body becomes love and the hand is restored. And as I told you, the two most important ones to Pamela, when I asked her were these mother's violent scenes and her littleness in the nightmare.

Cast of characters at the end of therapy, June, 1962: Pamela who says that, "Now I am different and I can never again be as I was before, who is no longer an oddity but feminine--to stand up to her mother--Pamela who has changed her life style, who plans to live alone soon.

Mother, who is more orderly in the house and who has much more respect for Pamela, who is even a little bit afraid of her, certainly more accepting of her. Mother, who is going to have to find either herself or another victim, or will consume herself.

Grandmother, now really dead--for the first time grandmother is dead, though she died nine years ago.

The family women, whom Pamela will use as a testing ground of her new independent body and whose bosoms no longer tower over her--the shelf - and whose "hermaphroditism" is now clear to Pamela, and which state she never accepted for herself all the time growing up.

The acrobatic teacher, who is now revealed as an exhibitionist and a sadist and a puppet in the grandmother's hands to excite herself by voyeurism.

The doctors, who worked for the psychotherapist, for Pamela's health--tests and check ups and so forth.

Dr. X, who had the perception, the integrity and a broad view, to call in the aid of doctors when needed, and to utilize them in therapy, and to be in session by session in conference with every single doctor and therapist.

Two other characters: Pamela's short lived lover, Olcott, who found his identity in the studio when he visited it--that is, in Pamela's dream. In one of her last sessions, she said, "He was here, right in this room, the studio--it was a lovely dream." Pamela's body had become feminine and the studio had become love.

And the father, to help Pamela to find him in the man she marries. This is the end, except that as in all therapy that works, the end was the beginning of a better life.

Any questions?

End of Tape

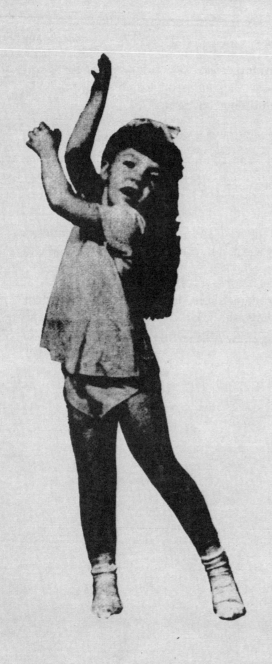

THE CHILD'S WORLD

Its Relation to Dance Pedagogy

a series of articles by

Blanche Evan

THE CHILD'S WORLD
Its Relation
to Dance
Pedagogy
a series of articles by

Blanche Evan

Preface

The ten articles that comprise "The Child's World" Its Relation to Dance Pedagogy" appear in this reprint in their original content. These article have long been out of print. It is hoped that this reprint will fill the requests of teachers and students who have continued to ask for them since their first publication by Dance Magazine.

Although my work and its literary expression have naturally grown in the intervening years, with especial concentration on the therapeutic aspects of Creative Dance, yet I feel these essays need not be revised. In an unpublished manuscript written before 1940 I stated that my primary concern in teaching would be

"first, the human being; second, a better person toward a better world"

These two tenets continue to guide my work and support the basic substance of these articles

Spring, 1964

New York City

PREFACE

The ten articles that comprise "The Child's World: Its Relation to Dance Pedagogy" appear in this reprint in their original content. These articles have long been out of print. It is hoped that this reprint will fill the requests of teachers and students who have continued to ask for them since their first publication by Dance Magazine.

Although my work and its literary expression have naturally grown in the intervening years, with especial concentration on the therapeutic aspects of Creative Dance, yet I feel these essays need not be revised. In an unpublished manuscript written before 1940 I stated that my primary concern in teaching would be

"first, the human being; second, a better person toward a better world"

These two tenets continue to guide my work and support the basic substance of these articles.

Spring, 1964
New York City

The Journal of

Pastoral Counseling

Volume V   Spring-Summer 1970   Number 1

"...THE LEAST MOVEMENT OF THE BODY"
BY BLANCHE EVAN[*]

The cliffs of Monhegan rise sheer from the Atlantic, their vertical strength balanced both by the horizontal landscape they protect and the undulating force of the sea they face. Their material substance seems to soften as they reflect the light of the sun and moon, to harden when they stand adamant and unaffected by the beating of the relentless rain. The rock comes alive to us as we respond to it. The body of the hills fuses with the spirituality we impart on them by way of our response and our love for these hills of Monhegan.[1]

In the summer of 1946 I sat on these cliffs with a young refugee minister from war-torn Hungary. I told him how these sea-borne hills seemed to be a symbol of my art, the Dance--the art of fusion of the physical with the spiritual: "...in the Dance the boundaries between body and soul are effaced. The body moves itself spiritually, the spirit bodily" says Van Der Leeuw in his extraordinary book *The Holy in Art.*[2] He tried to understand. He spoke to me of his personal growth in his pastoral education, his mind reaching beyond the clerical training he had had in Hungary and his body heretically in conflict with his position of minister.

Ten years later in 1956 when I studied at the Alfred Adler Institute of Individual Psychology in New York there were, along with the 15 or so psychotherapists taking the Course, four laymen: a social worker, a minister, a rabbi, and myself, a dance professional. Ten years after that when I had organically grown from dancer to dance therapist, I enrolled in my dance therapy session several rabbis, daughters of ministers, wives of rabbis and a nun. This year one of my students has as her counselor a clergyman who treats her in offices outside the church, (the American Foundation of Religion and Psychiatry). She sought out the Dance Therapy Centre on her own. Her counselor barely tolerated her idea, certainly lent no support. His ignorance of body movement--Dance therapy--added to his own "body" prejudices caused him to be cynical of its value. My student said: "He's a wonderful therapist for me but I know he has to overcome his background prejudices."

It made me recall my brilliant minister friend so tormented with his learned attitudes to the body.

The pastoral counselor even more so than the non-pastoral counselor has to face up to and undergo a change in these attitudes and to his own body as he in all honesty makes use of the area of body movement and Dance therapy, so vital and so appropriate in treatment of current neurosis.

"Enmity Between Dance and Religion"

This is the title of Van der Leeuw's book. He writes, "But almost from the very beginning, Christianity has been the outspoken enemy of the body..."

In the early centuries of our country, American Puritan hostility to Dance was raging.[3]

"The church" writes Van der Leeuw, "sings, paints, and builds, but it does not dance; or at least it does so no longer. Once it did dance,[4] and occasionally, in some hidden corner, it still does." Any pastoral counselor interested in this subject should read Chapter V, "The Roman Christian Church," of Lincoln Kirstein's *Dance*, Putnam, New York, 1935; also the Van der Leeuw book often referred to in this article; and many chapters (with an extraordinary bibliography) in *The Art of the Rhythmic Choir*, by Margaret Palmer Fisk, Harper & Bros., New York, 1950. These books contain historical material that describe both the "Enmity between Dance and Religion" and the "Unity of Dance and Religion." References include the numerous Old Testament pro-Dance pronouncements and the dances of David and other leaders; also the social structure *religious* dances: of celebration of the harvest and water-drawing.

"The Life of Man is the Life of a Moving Being"[5]

The human body functions only by movement: the inner moving process of muscles, joints, nerves, glands, and the five senses live by movement. Mentality and spirituality derive from a body in motion internally and of necessity externally. Adler said this succinctly:

"We can ascertain then in the very beginning that the development of the psychic life is connected with movement, and that the evolution and progress of all those things which are accomplished by the soul are conditioned by the free movability of the organism. This movability stimulates, promotes, and requires an always greater intensification of the psychic life. Imagine an individual to whom we have predicted every movement, and we can conceive of his psychic life as at a standstill.

"There is a strict corollary between movement and psychic life. In the evolution of the psychic life, therefore, we must consider everything which is connected with movement. We see that both mind and body are expression of life: they are parts of the whole of life. And we begin to understand their reciprocal relations in that whole. *The life of man is the life of a moving being.*"[6]

Yes, "the life of man is the life of a moving being" but the typical urban body in the United States has ceased moving. Simultaneously mental illness--a gross *misnomer*--has been increasing at an alarming rate.

This is the machine age. Machine displaces human action. Formerly human work expended natural energy. Work demanded big and small muscle use. Work kept the blood circulating and increased the lung power. Work gave dignity and a reality to ego. These are only some of the ingredients that have now become a vacuum. (The hopeless urbanite replies "Just as well--what good to breathe in more polluted air." What a vicious cycle industrialization has spawned.) Enormous and small machines and "make life easier" gadgets deprive the human body of action necessary to health. Finally the adult's inclination to "no effort" is exploited by amoral business and advertising: "no need for the body to work--keep fit *without* exercise--use the vibrating belt," etc. No need for the person to DO, only to be done to. Depersonalization.

In addition to the more physical aspects, this replacement of work by the machine has had far reaching PSYCHOLOGICAL EFFECTS, ON AFFECTS, unknown to most therapists, even to those who refer patients with the request "help them release their tension and express their anger." Physical work is a great outlet for anger and aggression and their accompanying tension, *even when used symbolically in an action class*. Work energy is a socially acceptable sublimation and displacement for these feelings. To the private urban citizen to be civilized means to repress aggression and anger *with no active alternate supplied*. Yet the anger and aggression are there. Adrenalin is automatically produced in the body for action which "normally" results from these feelings.[7] With action repressed, the energy is diverted to different kinds of tension: rigidity at one extreme, apathy at the other. Every dance therapist is familiar with both psycho-physical states. The "head" takes over--how many of my referred patients come to sessions with headaches, leave without them--the brain wheels turn round and round, ironically in a machine-like way, the nerves work overtime to KEEP THE BODY FROM ACTION, hostilities store up until they come near to bursting and the media and professional sports take over offering a sick outlet of passive violence--"read all about it"--"see it on TV." The no-outlet energy for some becomes active-destructive violence, outwardly to the world and/or inwardly to one's self.

Finally an enormous amount of energy is used *to maintain self-defeating attitudes*. The human body loses its form, its grace, its power to express, and finally the natural NEED to express is stifled. ("I can't cry.") Body and spirit split and begin to atrophy; ego power shrinks to low self-esteem with an ineptness for both anger and love. In our dance therapy sessions those who cannot be strong in movement can neither be tender; those who cannot express love can neither dance anger. There may be millions of neurotics who fit diagnostic cabinets but *there are also millions of a nondescript nature who fit into the category of what the new age has done to the human being.*

"Older than all preached Gospels was this unpreached, inarticulate but ineradicable, forever-enduring Gospel: work, and therein well being." (Carlyle in *Past and Present.*)

Inaction and depression go hand in hand. Bleuler described the "melancholic triad consisting of depressive affect, inhibition of action and inhibition of thinking," Beck in *Depression* refers to "...a reduction in spontaneous activity."[8]

75% of the patients who come to me state verbally their need to express their long contained anger. We have many techniques for that, a few of them fairly simple: beating on a hassock, pounding a drum, transferring the drum action to body action without the drum, both heavy and staccato work actions simulating manual labor, can be done (except perhaps the drum) within the counselor's sessions in a small space. Pick out the action words in your patient's verbalization, and encourage him to put this action *word* into *action*. Go on from "I feel" into *doing* that feeling; from "I wish" into *moving* that fantasy. You don't need to know "how to dance" but you do need to *admit* to feeling the emotional substance of your words that demand action.

Aridity of feeling is seen in the frozen face of the neurotic. The mask presents an acceptable face to the world, a nothing non-committal expressionless expression. When a patient says "I don't feel anything" I suggest: MOVE and you may stir up feeling. Move your face, too." The mask conceals: "many patients conceal their unpleasant feelings behind a cheerful facade."[9] It is one of the most difficult immobilized areas to reach--it would seem to be the next to last physical defense that the patient will not relinquish. Perhaps because when the facial mask is discarded, the patient will no longer be able to say "I don't feel anything." The counselor can learn ways to help the patient relax the facial prison both with and without a mirror. To "make faces" is another way, not a game but an important part of freedom seeking.

I asked a patient how she washed her face. She threw water at it. We went to the wash basin and let the water run. She really spurted drop of water AT her face. She could not bear to touch her face *with her hands.*

Have you ever seen your patients' hands?

I had one referred patient who clenched his hands unconsciously every time he was overwhelmed with antagonism to his brother.[10]

The therapist can profitably learn to interpret hands. When advisable he can also learn ways to bring the hands of the patient out of listlessness to life, and out of tension to action. In recent experience, work with the hands was followed by voluntary verbalizations: of stifled aggression with attendant quilt; the secrecy of masturbation and recall of parental violence when the child had been "caught"; the shame of having "ugly" hands--"not beautiful like my sister's" followed by a long bitter story of sibling rivalry. And "washing" the hands--there are thousands of aspiring Lady Macbeths around.

Hands are used much in gestalt therapy. I have witnessed both the late Fritz Perls and an eclectic therapist at two different marathons using the hands of patients to symbolize specific conflicts in the patient. Very effectively too.

In the art of East Indian Dance the Mudras form a whole language of hand gesture communicating whole sentences of thoughts. Consciously and unconsciously in life and in art the hands speak.

The overall label is TENSION. The counselor can learn fairly simple exercises to give for relaxation, especially for the neck and head. Most people who attend the Dance Therapy Centre ask for relief in these areas. Perhaps you fear that the patient will be digressed from what is bothering him psychologically--not at all. If he had an infected pimple, you would suggest he go to a doctor and have the pus drained out, even though another pimple might appear. While a patient is going through therapy he still must live. Relief in the relaxation of muscular tension also opens up verbalization--certainly preferable in most cases to the passive tranquilizer pill.

Eyes: for the Therapist

The observation of, and the use of posture as an indicator of the patient's emotional problems form an important part of body movement and dance therapy.[11] If the therapist is to use these means of interpreting and working with the patient he really has to develop his eyes, add seeing to listening, seeing the patient in a new psycho-physical entity. And if he *sees* the patient, the seeing may become reciprocal--the patient is going to see him, he will be seen. What does the therapist's posture reveal? Has he himself seen it? As you sit and read this article, how are you sitting? What does your posture reveal to you?

Ears for the Patient: Self Sound

One of my most startling cases last season was the singer who sought treatment at the Dance Therapy Centre *because he had lost his singing voice.* His body movement and dance improvisations turned to childhood themes and recollections. I suggested adding humming to his movements which over a period of weeks grew to syllabic sounds. When his improvisation became very hostile to, as he explained, one of his parental figures, I suggested singing out his hostility. The word HATE was chosen. In gradual crescendo he emitted the most powerful song built on that word--the walls shook. He said it was the best singing he had ever done in his life. It freed him to return to his regular repertory, the lost voice in voice again.

Other means of self-sound for non-singer are clapping hands or rhythmically lightly slapping one's hands against parts of the body; also clapping with someone else's hands and clapping for someone who is dancing. The self-produced sounds seem to wake up the whole person in an immediate kind of way. The most difficult area is the production of throat and gut sounds related to the significance of the movement being expressed. In this area of self-sound the neurotic is repressed even more so than in moving the face.

I recall a set of parents who FOR PUNISHMENT rolled their infant daughter's carriage into the hallway WHEN SHE CRIED, and left her there alone. Who knows? "A baby tells all its secrets with its mouth, ...a mouth that seems always speaking silently or otherwise" (Millen Brand). If sound repression is enforced in infancy; and in childhood the patient has been disciplined "to speak when you are spoken to" and to "shut your mouth," etc, the whole trapped sound of the adult appears to be a logical outcome. To release this sound opens up the dammed up rancid waters of bitter frustration. Resistance to body movement is easier to break through than self-sound because, out of realistic necessity, the infant and child HAD to continue to move the body and could not be coerced as much into "stop moving" as into "be quiet."

It is perhaps relevant that the psychotic not only hears voices but feels free to emit screams and a flow of Joyceian language. He is also much more free in body movement and expression and more organized in rhythm than the neurotic. If we can make possible for the neurotic the opportunity to release body movement, sound and expression in addition to his verbalization, we might more effectively help forestall that day when he can no longer tolerate his immobilizations, when he comes near to "breakdown."

Outer Sound: An Accompaniment for Movement

Dance improvisation without or to music is a profound expression of the starved neurotic. In its simplest form it can be practised and conducted by private and group therapists, and executed by non-dancers. Especially to songs. Patients who suffer with maternal rejection never fail to react when they improvise to "Sometimes I Feel Like a Motherless Child" as sung by Marian Anderson or Dorothy Maynor. Spirituals of many kinds are easily available on recordings. Many of the songs of Miriam Makeba and Harry Belefonte are also easy to interpret in movement and mime. Their melodic words hit the patient with personal identification. Sealed tear ducts are pried open and made to flow. Last season several therapists asked me to conduct Dance therapy sessions with their groups to be immediately followed by verbalization with the attending group therapist. Among the successful themes I used for the dancing with appropriate music was that of adolescent stages of life. (The therapists were amazed at how much they learned about their patients by *watching* them, in a new kind of way different from always listening to them.)

The rock and roll teens may prefer songs from the musical HAIR to spirituals. If that takes the lid off their boiling self-defeat, why not? HAIR has some songs whose words are directly therapeutically valuable. There are also many *non* rock and roll teens in therapy. I am looking at a very dignified ad in the New York Times picturing such a girl. It is an apparel ad, and the copy reads:..."in the skirt that suggest *the body in motion,* even when it isn't." (Italics mine.)

From England there is a record called *A Man Dies*,[12] originally written for the teenagers of St. James' Presbyterian Church, Lockleaze, Bristol. It is an attempt to present the Bible story in the modern idiom--in the music and dancing which teenagers love so much and can do so well...written by Evan Hooper and Ernest Marvin, Minister of St. James...it combines satire, humor, and social comment with the Gospel story...Gospel simply means 'good news' and Liturgy, 'the work of the people.' Produced and seen latest version in 1964 at the Royal Albert Hall, London and on national network Television"." There are 26 songs with the reprise GENTLE CHRIST. One of the songs is a modern manger birth parallel; another, GO IT ALONE which ends "WE DIDN'T HAVE TO GO IT ALONE." The cover notes are very informative and descriptive of the church activities out of which *A Man Dies* came to being.

Listening

Music listening has far outgrown the purpose of "soothing the savage beast." For those adult patients who are experiencing great conflict in the area of their faith there is Leonard Bernstein's SYMPHONY No. 3, the KADDISH,[13] "dedicated to the Beloved Memory of John F. Kennedy." "The Kaddish, (Sanctification)...is the name of the prayer chanted for the dead."

It is a shocking and magnificent work. Excerpts: "Great God surely you who make peace on high/ Who manipulate clumsy galaxies/You who juggle a spaceful of suns/Bend light, spin moons.../

Surely you can handily supply/A touch of order here below/On this one, dazed speck/And let us say again...Amen/Always you have saluted me/With a rainbow, a raven, a plague, something./But now I see nothing./ This time you show me/ Nothing at all/ Ani Havazelet ha Sharon, the lily/ That man has picked and thrown away!/...tin god!/ Your bargain is tin! It crumples in my hand!/ And where is faith now--yours OR mine?/ ...There is nothing to dream./ Nowhere to go./ Nothing to know.../ Come back with me, to the Star of Regret/ Come back, Father, where dreaming is real/ and pain is possible--so possible You will have to believe it/ And in pain/ You will recognize your image at last/ Together we suffer, together exist/ And forever will recreate each other."

This music with text pierces the heart and jumps hurdles that the timid confused faith-doubting neurotic would take years to bring to the surface. "...strangely enough, there is not a single mention of death in the entire prayer. On the contrary, it uses the word Chaye or chaim, (life) three times. Far from being a threnody, the Kaddish is a compilation of paeans in praise of God..."

For a group tormented by religious doubts, a group therapy hour listening to this recording could be a very stimulating and cathartic experience. It might help one to find his own way on the road of nettles to and away from faith.

In our dance therapy sessions there are occasional requests for themes to express the students' or patients' conflicts in faith. This year one of these, a Jew, danced out some of this Symphony. She crashed with faith and eventually resolved the dance into a personal confrontation with her fear and ambivalence of and to the authority figures in her life. I also recall an orthodox Catholic student who swerved between suicide and becoming a nun who to other accompaniment danced "Temptations of St. Anthony." Her dance just ached to be handed, as on a platter, to her therapist.

There is another kind of inspirational listening, as listening, or for dance, for those in conflict with faith in the church or in man or in the very value of life itself. I refer to Mahler's second symphony, the "Resurrection."

Music in its own way, like movement, mime and self-sound, can act as a trigger and a wedge.

The Rhythmic Choir

There are surprising quotations in the reference works mentioned in this article, on dance in the Christian church: the fantasy of Machtild of Magdeburg in the thirteen century which she called THE FLOWING LIGHT OF GOD in which she relates her creation of a holy dance; and the nun's hymn, about 1440, which reads: "Let us all together on the road to heaven./ There, where joyous music rings, we shall with angels dance along,/ To the sweet heavenly strings."

That the church is no stranger to dance has been borne out in our own time by the work of Margaret Palmer Fisk. Herself a minister's wife, she was a great innovator in restoring Dance to meet the needs of the modern parishioner within the Church itself. She organized the "Rhythmic Choir" which was not a singing choir, but a body-movement-Dance group activity. A minister's wife says of the rhythms class Mrs. Fisk conducted: "The music started and I followed the movements. Then a miracle started to happen to me. The cold hard shell of me which years of sermons, conferences, prayers, poems, and all the other phases of ordinary worship had left untouched, crumbled into dust...As I stretched my arms to the side...the love of God flooded into my opened heart. Through the most unexpected phase...I found what I had come to find: God."[14]

Unknowingly, Mrs. Fisk probably became the first body-movement-Dance therapist for one kind of neurotic in America. She writes: "There is a serious need for training in the creative technique of the body-soul growth and health, for they are mutually helpful." It is amazing how people of different backgrounds and objectives suddenly meet on a common denominator level. I am not religiously oriented, yet here I find in Mrs. Fisk's book:[15] "The timid, tightly repressed individual comes to enjoy wide, flowing movements, learns to relax the jaw and hands, and feels at home with the group..."

As far back as 1919, in New York, an Episcopal rector, William Norman Guthrie, felt the need for training the body to express the spirit. "Our bodies," he said, "must become active means of projecting deep, creative ideals, so that we may become adequate vehicles--translucent to that imminent Life of the Creative God." St. Marks-in-the-Bowerie, on Second Avenue and 10th Street, New York, was his church from 1919-1938. "The rhythmic movements were called 'Eurhythmic Rituals' and used a combination of professional dancers and members of the congregation. About seven programs were given each year." In the 1920's Bird Larson of Columbia University staged these choreographed works for the church. "It was not long before leaders in Roman Catholic, Methodist, Presbyterian (and many other denominations), started to experiment in this art of the rhythmic choir or in the spiritual art of creative movement."

"Rev. Robert A. Storer, pastor of the First Parish Church, Unitarian, in Dorchester, Mass....wrote his B.D. thesis on 'The Dance as Sacred Ritual' in 1937...He experimented directly with motion choirs...His pioneer work has a reverence that has made it acceptable to 'conservative' New England...In 1949 he gave a two-hour lecture demonstration at Old South Church in Boston as part of a Lenten Institute sponsored by the Massachusetts Council of Churches."

Mrs. Fisk was not, nor ever intended to be, a counselor. However, her work certainly was therapeutic. She physicalized feelings that had been accepted as appropriate only to prayer, to talking, to singing. She too speaks of the adolescent and the use of music and gesture. The Fisk book is a generation away from the record and cover notes of *A Man Dies*, the English production referred to in this article. Both are valid.

Out of Touch

Bellevue Psychiatric has had volunteer dance therapists since the forties. Veteran's hospitals now employ them as well as many other institutions where total push programs are the objectives. The *psychotic* is programmed for movement, dance, and music therapy but the neurotic in private therapy or clinics fares less well. He has to seek it out on his own because only a minority of therapists make direct referrals. The field is relatively unknown and now is being confused with encounter and sensitivity groups neither of which derive from Dance.

The therapist who has had no personal experience in body therapy does not realize that non-verbal therapy can be an adjunct to, rather than a substitute for verbalization. The insights gained through movement channels *are* unique but seep back to feed and to free verbal communication. These gains are made through the medium of the patient with or without contact between prime and adjunctive therapist.

The founders of psychiatry wrote that body movement expressed the psyche: Freud, Adler, Reich, Kretschmer, and more recently Paul Schilder. Deprived of movement the psyche must suffer. Rehabilitation and total health cannot occur by further separating the feelings of the mind and the body but rather by REUNITING them. In our disjointed life, therapy entails more than changing attitudes or reconstructing the personality. To be more effective it should RESTORE that seed of UNITY the child experienced in pre-verbal stages of growth.[16] Again, from Van der Leeuw: "Yet we shall not go far astray if we see, in the continually growing demands which things of the body make upon our culture, an expression of the same spirit which, in psychology and philosophy, once more desires to view a man as a unity; not as a soul in an accidental body, but as a single organism whose deepest essence expresses itself as much in the least movement of the body as in speech or thought..the whole body can be an expression...of all that moves the person."[17]

In our daily life today the city tears apart sound, congeals movement, crushes the individual body in thick masses of bodies. It would indeed seem that "there is nothing fixed in the relationship of parts" (E. Mark Stern). The one ENTITY that still remains is the human body, more fixed than any other phenomenon. 50% of the referred patients who come to the Dance Therapy Centre whisper, at the interview, "I am out of touch with my body." Therapy limited to verbalization no longer fills this gap. In many instances the patient has not told the prime therapist about being "out of touch with his body" nor has the therapist ever asked his patient: "are you in touch with your body?"[18] If he did ask the question in most cases he would not be equipped to know what to do about it.

This is an indication of what Dance and body movement therapy are all about. Not alone better health OF the body, OR the mind, OR the feelings, but better PSYCHOPHYSICAL HEALTH. SOMA means BODY *not* SICK body. I should like to add to the concept of psychosomatic illness my own development concept of PSYCHOSOMATIC HEALTH.

To be out of touch with the body and to deal with this in body movement and dance therapy requires a deep level of professional study. A well known secular psychiatrist who attended one of our seminars put it to the discussants with disarming honesty: "The therapist is not in a position to deal with this because we have the same hangups with our bodies as do our patients."

To *incorporate* body movement--corpus-body--into therapy--there are various methods that relate to individual patient, therapist and dance therapist. For the pastoral counselor, in addition, there is the balancing out of personal credo as matured in pastoral training. Also there is no substitute for direct experience, and any counselor interested in applying this work needs to attend participating sessions in it.

No one asks the therapist nor the patient to become a dancer. Expressive movement like song are nature's gift. For a moment leave what you have already learned and look around you. Do you think that automation does not cause imbalance in the human system? Or that for man to step on the moon, literally, does not require a reorientation to space--in terms of human equilibrium? Or that to go around the world on "vacation" in a couple of days without getting up from your airplane seat does not need a time adjustment for the mere speck of the human being who has become so small in body compared to what is being done *for* him?

No. you do not have to be a dancer to make use of this work, but Dance leads the way. Dance is the one art that "projects the spirit of man through the body, the spirit fused with the body of motion outward into space and time."[19]

Freud, the Shrink

Unthinkable! How disrespectful! Just doesn't fit. Anachronism in reverse. His way was to expand not to contract the analysand.

Does it fit *you* to be labeled by your patient HEAD SHRINKER now cut down to SHRINK? How awful. Let's change it.

Repersonalization.

By way of reintegration of body, mind and spirit.

Reich says in *Character Analysis*: "In the dancer the main expressive movements derive from the total organism."

SUMMARY

This article has presented new concepts:

1. That the counselor recognizes the neuroses that *derive* from the society of NOW. Parents plus.

2. That the pastoral therapist add seeing to hearing--eyes to ears in the immediate counseling session.

3. That he develop movement, dance and music uses in the private and group therapy sessions, thus adding a new dimension to verbalization.

4. That he distinguish between what he can add to his own techniques, from the deeper approach available in the dance therapist's specialized place of work.

5. That the adjunct adds to but does not substitute for verbalization.

6. That there is an historical viewpoint both positive and negative in the Church in its relation to the body and to the art of Dance.

7. That to deny the increasing awareness on the part of the patient to his new psychophysical needs can only alienate the patient who today seems more and more determined to seek out and to find non-verbal adjunctive therapies: music, art, and, in this case, body movement and dance improvisation.

REACTION by Sister Patricia Pak-Poy, R.S.M., Convent of Mercy, Erindale, South Australia

Whether one accepts the human person as a body-spirit, or as merely a body, or as a psychophysical entity, one can hardly object to the concept of the dance as valid form of self-expression. Blanche Evan's exposition of dance therapy as an adjunct of psychotherapy and counseling is a positive statement about the vital role of the body in a person's self-integration and a plea for counselors to develop new ears, perhaps a fourth and a fifth, to help their patients by understanding them through their body-movement.

Miss Evan's comment that there has always been an opposition between dance and religion is valid insofar as all form of Christianity have repudiated excesses which have led to orgies of one kind or another, such as the Bacchanalia. The dichotomy of body and spirit, too, has led to the inhibition of the body as the inferior element in man, and a denial of its freedom lest it control the spirit.

However, modern man is more aware of the unifying function of the tension of the elements that make him a body-spirit. We accept this in accepting the significance of conventional gestures such as hand-shaking, waving and beckoning, yet somehow we hesitate about accepting spontaneous and free expression of the whole body. The ballet, folk dancing or ballroom dancing seem to be more acceptable forms, maybe because they are pre-patterned and in this way "controlled expression."

Interpretative and spontaneous dance can be more chaotic, it is true, but is, generally speaking, a better vehicle for self-expression and communication. Like play therapy, psychodrama and mime, it has great therapeutic potential and I would like to see this technique further developed by specialists, and in wider use among counselors who, as Miss Evan insists, must have participated themselves and have acquired some skill in the preparation of patients for this form of expressions (e.g. Laban's methodology), and at interpreting gesture and movement. The point is also well made that the dance is not a substitute for verbalization, but can be a help to the patient in his striving for full consciousness of his feelings and the verbalization of them. For the patient it is a step towards personal integration, and the counselor must recognize his own limitations with the use of this form of therapeutic expression, just as he must recognize his limitations as a pastoral counselor: he is not a psychotherapist. I would think that beginning counselors and "beginning patients" (i.e those beginning dance therapy) would be more at ease in a group than in one-to-one therapy or counseling. I think there is some validity in the generalization that modern man, at least in Western cultures, is "out of touch with his body" almost in the same way as he is "out of touch" with his feelings because society has required man to be un-emotive if he is to be manly and strong. Alternatively, he feels split into a body and spirit at war with each other, and he must search for reunification. He may find this resolution of tension in athletic or eurythmics or hatha yoga or in interpretive dance; or he may deny the split consciously or unconsciously, to the detriment of his wholeness.

Miss Evan's brief exposition on "self sound" describes a process which is important. One must be free to make sound. To me, dance alone is one form of expression, but dance to the accompaniment of one's own voice, with or without words, is a fuller expression of thought and emotion, and perhaps therapeutically more valuable. This is why I would have reservations about using such songs as *Sometimes I Feel Like a Motherless Child* as stimuli--the words direct the patients' thoughts and feelings too pointedly.

Outer sounds and accompaniment are important for setting the mood though care must be taken that the counselor does not manipulate the emotions of the patient by these means. There may also be a need for a framework, such as the gospel story in *A Man Dies*. I think the value of this particular work is not so much in the dance or music as therapy, as in the therapeutic and educational effect on the performers as they work with a group to express religious understanding in music, speech and dance of their own idiom. In the performance I saw of this play, there was certainly emotional release both for the players and the audience, and no doubt there were therapeutic gains, but the play was not primarily designed as therapy. However, tapping the therapeutic potential of such a work is legitimate, and I agree with Miss Evan that there are many forms of activity which should be explored for what they can contribute directly to therapy. Creative listening to music is one form; dance is another. Even as adjuncts to therapy or counseling, they will not suit every counselor nor every client, but those who have an affinity for these forms are to be encouraged to explore further this new form of helping others strengthen their grasp on lived life.

The beautiful truth burst upon my mind—I felt that there were invisible lines stretched between my spirit and the spirits of others.   —Helen Keller

FOOTNOTES

1. The Hills of Monhegan Island off the coast of Maine, U.S.A.

2. *Sacred and Profane Beauty: The Holy in Art*, by Garardus Van Der Leeuw, Holt, Rinehart and Winston, New York, 1963. "A poet, musician, man of the Church and Minister of Education."

3. See *The Puritan and Fair Terpsichore*, by A.C. Cole, Mississippi Valley Historical Review, vol. XXIX, No. 1, June 1942.

4. "The Dance in Shaker Ritual," by E.D. Andrews, in *Chronicles of the American Dance*, edited by P. Magriel, Henry Holt, N.Y., 1948.

5. *Understanding Human Nature*, by Alfred Adler.

6. *What Life Should Mean to You*, by Alfred Adler.

7. *Bodily Changes in Pain, Hunger, Fear and Rage*, by Dr. Walter B. Cannon, T. Branford Co., Boston, 1953.

8. *Depression*, by A.T. Beck, M.D. Harper and Rowe, 1967.

9. See film *Life is Movement*, distributed by Dance Therapy Centre, 5 W. 20 St, N.Y. 10011.

10. "Hands grip first in the embryo and sometimes are born with scratches from their own nails," *A Child is Born*, by A. Ingelman-Sundberg, Delacorte Press, N.Y.C., 1965.

11. Read "Article IV. A Technique for the City," in *The Child's World: Its Relation to Dance Pedagogy*, by Blanche Evan, pub. Dance Therapy Centre.

12. See *Baltimore Sunday Sun*, January 12, 1968, *Family*, by Barbara Rowes.

13. *A Man Dies*. EMI Records Ltd., Hayes, Middlesex, Eng. No. 33SX1609.

14. Columbia KL 6005.

15. *The Art of the Rhythmic Choir*, by Margaret P. Fisk, Harper and Brothers, 1950.

16. Fisk: *Ibid.*

17. See *The Child's World* (article II *ibid.*).

18. Van Der Leeuw, *ibid.*

19. The Reichian therapies certainly are the exception.

20. *The Dancer of Pompeii*, by Blanche Evan, Dance Magazine, March 1952.

the fog, the moon, the sun, and a Pathway to Dance/Movement Therapy
by Blanche Evan

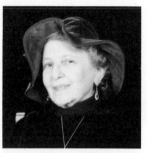

Blanche Evan

Sedona is becoming a place of urban interests in the arts in ways that complement its extraordinary rural setting. Many artists are brought in to perform and exhibit here. The various art centers offer fine instruction in the arts and crafts.

The use of the arts as therapy is relatively new in the United States and relatively unknown. This series of articles will deal exclusively with Dance/Movement Therapy in relation to the urban adult. It will point up the difference between "therapeutic" and "therapy".

Why here? Because Sedona people cherish freedom and Dance/Movement Therapy offers one vital means to free and unify YOUR total self.

Blanche Evan chose to dedicate her life to Dance when she was nine years old. She has never deviated. She studied many forms of art but concentrated mainly on Creative Dance. She has been performer, choreographer, author, teacher, and, since 1958, a pioneer in Dance and Body Movement therapy.

She is now a resident of Sedona and hopes to extend her activity to include the town which is now her home.

The grey mist and fog-shapes cover the red rocks of Sedona. As they drift, the proud look of centuries is revealed: the Cathedral Rocks, the Courthouse formations and the more plebeian Coffee Pot. (Man has a driving anthropomorphic need to identify with the wonders of nature by means of his own appellations.) The rain pours down creating gullies and little lakes, the brick red soil sucking up this long absent nourishment. The lover of Sedona does not complain. Last night the moon cast a pervasive glow while the coyotes barked their own response to the sky. And then suddenly, having concealed its warmth for days, the sun emerges, the wetness and the drought are forgotten, buds open and new seeds are planted.

Many adults live in Sedona to find peace, to rest from the pressures of the past, including twenty wild years of the "flower children". We are pleased with the rural quaintness of our town with the fast disappearing methods of P.O. Box No. at the post office, of the streets without known names and our house fronts without numbers (even though our guests cannot easily find us when they visit). People come from everywhere. License plates show states from every area in the United states. Those who remain here keep in touch through global media. Yet, we are spared the brunt of the terrorist and the visible decay of the big cities which we once considered "home". We have finally picked up and fled from the *social neuroses:* violence, greed, drugs, power drive, etc. The sensitive person hopes that the move will also abate the stress of tenacious personal problems. There is still the desire to achieve more positive values, to transmute confusion into will and insight, supported by the strength and beauty of the natural environment of Sedona.

When I entered the profession of Dance therapy I designated this kind of client as the "normal neurotic": the prevalent person who functions but without adequate fulfillment. Conflict assumes gargantuan proportion. The relentless persistent doubt of "WHO AM I" continues to plague this person. How can I be "they" and "them" and "that" when I want to be merely myself. Merely? One of the most difficult knots to untangle in therapy is GUILT: particularly the guilt that has accrued in one's lifetime for having allowed one's own potential to be squashed, ridiculed, isolated, until the shout became barely audible and the whisper most often choked into a sob.

We can't live it all over again, but we can live more fully, more creatively. We can reshape the repressions enforced in childhood: "don't run, you'll fall; don't swim, you'll drown; don't play in the snow, you'll catch pneumonia." Always the negative. On another level, "never

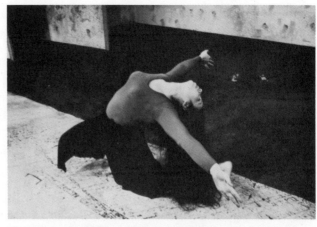

Final movement in a dance in which true artistry and true therapy are combined into a total experience. From Blanche Evan's film, "Life is Movement". *Film photo by A. Marks, courtesy of the Author.*

mind your feelings - just behave". The child's body grows despite this, lacking grace and without self-confidence. Later, the attempts to conceal this with garments and adornments leave the body itself unmotivated. Spontaneity rigidifies.

Nature's mechanism to maintain psychophysical health relies on movement. Dance/Movement Therapy, of course, is based on the body in actual movement. Not just any standard exercise, but movement which through concentration and guidance evokes from within, a movement based on stifled feeling - a movement that expresses your past, your present and at times your future. YOU move according to your individual structure, function, social mores, and habit. No one can move as you do because no one equates your unique totality. Out of your individuality you can create movement just as a novice can pick up a piece of chalk and draw or a brush with colors and paint.

The first fundamental change is the awakening that YOU HAVE THE RIGHT TO FEEL, TO OPEN UP and to express yourself as YOU rather than to be a mouthpiece for social setups of behavior that inwardly do not conform to your desired personality. In the process of therapy you have the acceptance by the therapist without censorship. "OUTLET" is a process of catharsis. It is therapeutic without necessarily being therapy. Therapy means growth and change and personal SELF-acceptance. It is diagnostic. Diagnosis is not abstract nor a copy of one school of psychotherapy or another.

How you see yourself - that is called "body image"; "body image" is not a stone fossil. You can learn to change it with will, with a sharpening of all your senses. Changing a body image can be tantamount to having the courage to wear a different hair-do, or to stop confiding in people to gain their "sympathy" when in truth they don't care. Seeking sympathy is often a tactic for diverting from the problem, a defense against facing up to it.

A body changes many times in one day in different situations. Which do you want, which are a burden that you can dispense with? How? Can you replace the pressure put on you by others (whose business it is not) by your own self-action? Can you stand on your own two feet? Can you arrive at a basic body image that *you* approve of? Can you expand it, change it when you want to? Do you have the imagination and the will to effect this? Can you develop what you lack? You *can* create your own body image and discard what has become a burden. This too is a process in learning the value of yourself and how to use it.

We speak of Dance/Movement therapy as a *psychophysical* process. At times the more physical components predominate, at other times the physical, the mind, the spirit. They interact in a process of liberation.

Dr. Alfred Adler, psychiatrist, (who contributed to his field the "inferiority complex", "life style" and many other important clarifications) wrote in his book *Understanding Human Nature:*

"There is a strict corollary between movement and psychic life...In the evolution of the psychic life, therefore, we must consider everything which is connected with movement...the evolution and progress of all those things which are accomplished by the soul are conditioned by the free movability of the organism. This movability stimulates, promotes, and requires an always greater intensification of the psychic life...Imagine an individual to whom we have predicated every movement and we can conceive of his psychic life as at a standstill."

Dance Therapy is only twenty-five years old in this country. It came into being at a time when the public was (and still is) entranced with the exquisite perfectionism of the visiting European ballet companies, which offered a super aesthetic experience to the observer. This time span also included the glamour period of Hollywood, the happy ending, the forever-smile of advertising, and the omnivorous capacity of the American audience *to look at* rather than *to do.* The layman judged the amateur's gratification as something to be ashamed of rather than what it is, something human, natural, and self-vindicating.

Then came the great American dancer, Isadora Duncan, who also rebelled against formalism. She created her own forms; she danced on all space levels, almost into the ground as well as on it. Rather than dancing stories or plots or rituals, she expressed her own feeling through the Dance. She was indeed Terpsichore's child. She even influenced the great Russian Ballet. Through the medium of her performance she spread freedom throughout America and Europe. *She made individual creative movement legitimate.* (She was not interested in the use of Dance as a medium of therapy.)

In its nascent stages, Dance Therapy was conceived as an *adjunctive* form: that is, we expected it to proceed according to the advices of a verbal therapist and in relation to the systems of therapy known as Freudian, Jungian, etc. In my own experience I learned eventually that the *channel* of body movement on a creative level of therapy was, and is, just as unknown to most psychotherapists as to the general public. As Dr. X said to me after one of my demonstrations, "we have the same hang-ups bodywise as our clients - how can we supervise you?" Each case is different. Some clients need both verbal and dance/movement therapy. Some cannot overcome their resistance to movement and do better with the verbal. I do believe in WORD. That is why I finally evolved my designation as "Dance/Movement/Word therapist". I am alerted to their use, interchangeably. In these years of practise, the many people who have become more free and more responsible to themselves and in some way to the world - these clients have proven that "Dance/Movement/Word" therapy can be a prime therapy.

When I first moved to Sedona my friends brought me a beautiful young tree. Not too long after, the leaves fell off - and it seemed dead. It was very sad. However, when Jan came and cleared the lawn of truly dead debris, she said "No, I'm not sure it is dead. I shall trim it down, cut off and throw away what IS dead; I shall give it tremendous nourishment for a while." Low and behold! The little nodules of life are appearing, new tender leaves are pushing their way through - out of their protective darkness into the light, the pure air of Sedona.

What Is there in you can move, can act, can renew, can live. In a Chinese poem, I find this line: "The muddy waters may yet become clear".

Source SEDONA LIFE March, 1978

the tree, the spine,
and the Myth of Posture
by Blanche Evan

"The Myth of Posture" and "Pathway to Dance/Movement Therapy" (March issue, *Sedona Life*) are not intended as simplistic reductions of people's problems. These articles do *not* represent belief in do-it-yourself programs without professional communication. Nonetheless, if your coat is buttoned up too tightly, only you can open it; only YOU can instigate action-for-change.

Posture is a psychophysical phenomenon. Among other factors, it is a culmination of cultural and environmental characteristics of where you live; of shifting tensions, frustrations and satisfactions; of climate and the evolution of chronological age. Posture is also the repository of trauma. Your posture is your story from prenatality to this moment of reading. Powerful. Yet we can gather the aggregate postural memory and put it through the sieve of maturity in order to become a liberated postural person of NOW.

COMMON MISCONCEPTIONS OF POSTURE ARE:

1. That posture is a pose rather than an organic manifestation.

2. That posture is an absolute - it is not: i.e., it is subject to tension and apathy from day to day.

3. That posture relates only to the standing position. No - it is also how you sit and lie down.

4. That posture is an accessory to put on and take off. No. Only if you are adept at "acting" what you pretend to feel.

5. That all exercises are appropriate to effect change. No; this is not the case.

6. That the main objective of posture is to appear in a way that society approves. This is practiced by many people, but basically, posture relates to health, the physiologic structure of the human anatomy, and to particular idiosyncracies.

Man is the only mammal that has achieved a vertical posture that stands at approximately a 90 degree angle to the base. There are theories that many of our illnesses are caused by the effort to maintain this verticality.

American Indian parents begin to condition the body for this upright spine by placing and carrying the infant on a straight cradle-board of wood. The American manufacturers distort this traditional health custom into a gimmick of *convenience* for the PARENT: a synthetic shapeless collapsible bag carrier placed on the back of the parent in which the little babybody is strapped into roundness, as if the child were still an embryo. An adult simulates this when he sits slumped in a chair, reading, eating, etc. - the abdominal area squeezing the chest, home of the heart and lungs. In ignorance of the body, the neurotic client who habitually distorts body position complains of "shallow breathing" as if this were only a *psychic* symptom. Bubbles, the escaped baby hippo in California weighing two tons, died recently because when they caught up with and tranquilized her, her large hippo abdomen pressed so tightly against her lungs that she expired.

In human posture, the central core is the spine: 24 moveable vertebrae with a small inflexible tail bone at the end and the head attached at the top. (Through the spine flows rivers of nerves.) The spine is vertical but not straight as a ruler. In fact, it is shaped in an S curve with two *natural* curves: a small one in the neck (cervical) and a large one between waist and pelvis (lumbar). Both curves arc toward the front making the spine a strong, balanced, flexible ladder.

Postural changes occur from the moment of birth until death. The normal baby of two has a bulging belly and a deep lumbar curve which by the age of four has considerably lessened. By preadolescence, there is more length top to bottom and less width front to back. In adulthood, if the two natural spinal curves have remained exaggerated, the causes may be: structure (born with that tendency); illness (polio); habit (influenced by inertia); social standards (looks more sexy); trauma which settled into a fixed stance. ALL THESE ARE OPEN TO REMEDIAL REHABILITATION. EFFECTIVE REHABILITATION IS PSYCHOPHYSICAL.

In terms of postural mechanics, it is essential to understand that bones grow until 17 to 20 years, but they cannot move. They *are* moved into placements by the attached muscles. *Alignment* is the maintenance of bones in their proper perpendicular relationship to each other, which in turn assures an expanded chest and correctly placed pelvic tilt.

Many tall Americans stand badly because their muscles fail to support the long bones. Muscles gain strength and resiliency through use both in daily function and in exercise. In medical healing there has been a switch from passive immobility of the patient to active moving. If your work day includes push and pull, lifting, lowering, reaching, etc. your muscles are working. If in addition you attend an exercise class or Dance class, and a sports activity, all the better because you are supplementing the daily functional use of muscles. If you are sedentary most of the day and ride in your car the rest of the time, you are really begging for trouble as age approaches.

In *alignment* the total spinal structure is *upward* with the head poised, the limbs not dangly but connecting with aliveness to the torso. Each leg forms a triangle from hip socket down to the centered power of the ankle.

Please look down. If your ankles are leaning *in* (pronation) or *out* (supination) try to set them in the middle; your body cannot be aligned on a crooked base. Your feet are not roller skates to get you "there". In fact, to do that they have to be strong enough *to stand on*.

In a person weighing 150 lbs., according to Dr. B. Mensendieck, the feet weigh 3 lbs each - 6 pounds to carry 144 pounds! If they are not centered they may well throw the spine off; many back pains are relieved by foot (and shoe) therapy.

When I work with clients on posture, we start with the feet, just as the seed starts with roots - the flower and the fruit come last.

From the feet to the *head*: Only 7 limber cervical vertebrae hold up the ten pound head-weight in that person of 150 pounds. The *greatest conflict* in the contemporary American neurotic adult is that this 10 lb. weight "thinks" that the head is more important than the 140 pounds under it.

We are known as "a head culture". In Dance/Movement therapy the client *experiences* that the "head" cannot dominate in isolation. As long as the person disregards attachment and relationship among head, body and feelings, the unit of self will be split. A client put it this way: "I don't know what's my body, what's my mind - I am a walking mind". *As if body existed from the neck down! The physical* split is clear: only by continuous unblocked flow of blood circulation from heart to head can your brain receive the oxygen crucial to health. In a more caring society the heart would rule physically more than or as much as the head psychically. Oxygen would be esteemed as life giver the way the Incas revered the Sun. I am talking of today, of us, of pollution, of drug abuse, of our inflated intellects, of body ignorance, of the split between body, mind, and feelings. This schism is fashionable: the head is pure, the feelings impure, the action condemnatory, and the body guilt ridden.

The placement of the head in *alignment* is in a vertical line above the shoulders. You can place it there, but to keep it there you need to USE neck freedom: to *see* all around, to see *where* you are, where you are going, to look at people and the world, to look *through*, to hear *in* from without, to open the channels of the sense lodged *in the head*, and to give up the monotony of heavy head hanging: looking at the floor rather than the earth.

Why do I mention a "tree" in the title of this article? Because posture is symbolically related to a tree, The trunk is upward; the branches do not drop, but bend, supported by the trunk's strength even when it grows in an angle; it secures its branches -the branches, their leaves, flowers and fruit. Motion caused by the wind is supported by the strong central trunk, much as the arms and legs of man are supported by the torso.

Even a frail flower can withstand attack because, unseen by the human eye, the tendrils and the roots are working underneath the soil to hold the stem and give it support. Nature knew that to grow upward and maintain balance roots had to grow *down*.

In life we say "get your feet on the ground": pushing down for foundation from which one can rise up, spring up, descend down, forward or back, at will. The space of your own body can command the space around it. We cannot fly, yet numerous clients *want* to without the effort downward, just as others want to become invisible rather than to confront. Fantasy overrules reality. To go up *depends* on "down" aliveness. (A dancer who jumps high confirms this.) The soles of the feet are transmitters. The dark side of downness occurs when there is a break in the longitudinal message. Lacking this support, the body weight becomes too much for spinal verticality to master.

Call this downward pull "gravity", but then don't name it - better call it "being pulled down", sinking, discouragement, leading to defeat and symbolically to death, a dread anxiety. Some people are able to stretch out on the floor to rest. Others appear to be getting under it or fighting the fear of being sucked into it. A healthy animal resting in various positions can at any moment spring to its feet or stretch out fully, or up and away to run and play. In contrast, if you watch an adult (someone else or yourself) go from one space level to another, you see that the great desire is *not* to move but to abide by inertia. There is little instinctual grace left to shift from down to up or vice versa.

The insecurity of the adult who spends most of his total energy *down* with abdominal bulge, over-curved lumbar spine (lordosis) over-rounded shoulder girdle (kyphosis) is obviously out of alignment with himself. Shift from torso to eyes and you will see that his eyes also reflect lethargy, a hiding from the world, a lack of confrontation; the "where to go", the look of abandonment.

To change posture means that you *want* to be upright in stance, to forego postural fixations of childhood and the stubbornness of neurosis, to feel worthy enough to occupy and to command the space in which you move. IT IS THE ONLY SPACE YOU HAVE. It is granted you by nature. This does not forego natural moods or dips from high to low. Even in real depression, psychologists now agree in recommending movement as an integral part of therapy. Posture in each individual amounts to how he is coping with inertia. "Energy" to cope is mostly forward and upward with grounding downward.

HOW TO START: Stop thinking about how you look to others posturally (here is a tie-up with body image); transfer your concern to how your feelings are governing your stance. *Connect* feelings with posture.

Engage in exercise necessary in reshaping the muscles to hold your bones where needed. Carry over your efforts to daily living. Change the word "posture" to *"postures"* and become aware of the emotional content of them. Above all, if you have been a victim of nagging to "stand up straight", replace this with deeper meanings in your stance. Connect physical and psychical. Enlarge your space image by a new cognizance that posture is the encapsulation that comports you through the world space surrounding your body. You change the landscape or the road in which you stand or walk.

How to change posture? - By according to it a motive: to live man's domain in vertical stance; to move freely and expressively. Through will, insight, work and true pride to enjoy Nature's dispensation of being built, uniquely, as a human being.

Source — SEDONA LIFE APRIL MAY, 1978

Jagged Tensions
and the Flow
of
Dance/Movement Therapy

By Blanche Evan

Blanche Evan is the pioneer in Dance/Movement Therapy as applied to the "normal neurotic"--that is, the person who functions, but without adequate fulfillment. At the vanguard of a relatively new science, Ms. Evan utilizes dance and movement as practical therapy, a practice which is relatively unknown in the United States.

In Dance/Movement Therapy, many areas of neuroses are defined as a combination of psychological and physical elements, becoming a psychological phenomenon. And likewise, a similarly integrated therapy is often the solution.

For a more definitive introduction to Dance/Movement Therapy, please refer to Blanche Evan's earlier articles which appeared in Vol. III, No. 2 and No. 3, Sedona Life.

(Part one of two parts)

Tension...Rigidity...Relaxation...Apathy...Intensity...Resilience...

These words signify a multitude of meanings unrealized by people who suffer with tension and who need relaxation. In contemporary society, there are so many approaches to these conditions that many adults wander from one group to another seeking answers. The groups vary from the mystical to plain exercise, from short term workshops to extended time. Rarely are the participants given a perspective on the body itself or on ways a person can (and should be) responsible for mastering personal tension in the 24-hour day.

Recreation as relief is a blessing at times, but it is also a stopgap to insight and change. It never reaches depths of causes and cures; nor does it reckon with the inescapable dominance of individual personality and character.

This article will attempt to be practical about these matters and to clarify some of the psychological issues related to their body mechanisms.

Despite popular generalities, tension is not always destructive; it can be positive when it *is* functional and dynamic; i.e. when you face a *must* situation, tension can speed up your resources to advantage. Habitual tension, however, *is* destructive. *Merciless tension* can lead to *rigidity* in body, mind and spirit. *Relaxation* is negative when it is neighbor to *apathy*; whereas controlled relaxation is synonymous with *resiliency*. *Intensity* is neither tension nor relaxation. It is the force of feeling.

Twelve noon. Two office workers dashed out into the street, rushed to the deli, stood in line at the counter, paid the cashier, sat down opposite each other straining to hear their conversation amidst the clatter of dishes, tried to hold their breath until the smell of chlorine on the waiter's cloth had been absorbed into the already foul air, ate their food, drank their cokes, walked to the park for the last 15 minutes of lunch time.

"Look at that old woman," one said, "she looks as if her face would crack if she smiled."

"She's not old," her companion differed, "not more than 40, I'd wager. That mask-like face looks like concrete. She's rigid, not old."

Tension. The nerves assaulted. The digestive system churning. Social contact accelerated beyond communication. Body rhythm erratic. Exhaustion deferred.

On arriving home, one of the two turned on the TV with the sound up loud and watched a violent program which eased her own tension. The other, in her own apartment, collapsed into a disinterested miasma of "so what." Tension and Apathy. The tense person has a better chance of survival. The apathetic one has given up, given in, feels like a depleted bag.

A passing apathy is *not* depression, no more than is sadness. It is a let-down. It is not peace but temporary obliteration.

Both of these workers need rest. Rest is sought, though not always achieved, by distraction, by change of tempo, by environment, by sleep, by love, by a warm bath, by nutritious and enjoyable food, by a pill, by massage, etc. The purpose of rest is to enable the over contracted muscles and the frayed nerves to regain function, and for the circulation to become stabilized. The toxins leave the body. Ideally, the mind, the feeling and the body renew their contiguity.

It is necessary to find a new clarity for overused words. Tension and relaxation are now common words. Their components are less known: *contraction, expansion, stretch, intensity, rigidity,* and *spasm.*

CONTRACTION AND EXPANSION

In order to touch your hand to your shoulder, your elbow must bend. This action is made possible by the contraction of the biceps and other muscles in the arm. When in use, a *contracting* muscle becomes short and thick. When you straighten the arm the *same muscles* changes its shape to become longer in expansion. Muscles are elastic. When you elongate the muscle fibers more than they are used to, you are in a state of stretch. If you *overstretch*, injury is likely to occur.

If the elbow bend is for a small light action, the contraction required is small; if it is for a weighty movement, the contraction has to be stronger, and the muscle will be thicker. If, however, you load the muscle with more contraction than it need for the task, you create nervous tension. False contractions do not organically depend upon each other,

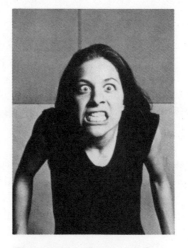
The tension of near-madness...
Photo by M. Swope

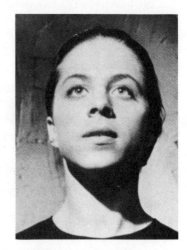
... and beautiful repose
Photo by A. Marks

but they have arisen at a feeling point and have been artificially maintained out of habit. False contraction stops movement, and like a tourniquet, stops circulation.

When contraction remains unyielding, *spasm* may occur. Then your joint actions are very stiff, and you are heading for a state of rigidity. Rigidity, however, is not paralysis.

INTENSITY

If you bend the elbow to do an expressive movement, *you* measure and control the amount of contraction beyond the functional need in the muscle. You decide the force you want for your expression, and your gesture is filled with any degree of strength you choose. You are also free to add force to a muscle in contraction or in expansion purely for dramatic emphasis. Spontaneous people do this many times in a day in speech, gesture, and even in casual contact. Actors and singers project largely through their dynamic range, and dancers are totally involved second by second in adding and diminishing force (intensity) to their muscles for dramatic emphasis.

That state in which muscles contract and expand according to function and expressive need without premeditation, I name RESILIENCY. It is the secret of body harmony in action. Lack of resiliency in major joints affects the whole body. For instance, if the knee joints are tight, the passage of continuous movement through the body is destroyed, no matter how limber the spine may be. Knee restraint - very prevalent.

BOTH OVERT AND SUBTLE TENSION

LEGITIMATE TENSION

A *stimulus to work;* as in meeting a deadline

anticipation

excitement

pre-performance "butterflies"

Fear:

real fear

phobic fear

vague anxiety fear

traumatic incident

Pain:

Swelling tissue

Nerves pressing on bones or being pressed on pinched nerve

arthritic pain

tooth-ache

other diseases

Deep distraught pain, as in loss of a loved one

DESTRUCTIVE TENSIONS

Among the fourteen examples that follow, there are many destructive tensions that exist in what I term "the 24-hour day", tensions which people accept as inevitable. Actually, with consciousness and will, the person can learn to be responsible for the quantity and specificity of the personal tension which he or she inflicts upon the self and others.

Tension beyond the individual's tolerance of stress leads to breakdown. If you *overwind* a watch, the motor stops. When a jar is filled to the top with water, one extra pebble placed in it will cause it to overflow

1. *Repression:* to withhold expression of feelings; *the work of bottling up the feelings*. I heard this on a bus: "I had to muster all my energy not to explode." If you keep the lid at least somewhat off the vessel, the steam has an outlet which will prevent over-flow. Tension is less damaging if let out along the way in small ways or large cathartic methods, than if it is contained until *explosion* occurs.

The tension of repressed love is common: "I love him, but I can't say to him 'I love you'." When you hold back expression of emotion, the emotion eventually stagnates. Your fear of life concentrates in your muscles.

Personality Tensions:

2. The tension of the drive to *overcontrol*.

3. The *pretense tension* of the (false) martyr.

4. *Tension that corrodes:* The corrosion of Envy.

5. The tenacious fantasy of *perfectionism* which encourages procrastination because of impossibility of attainment, with its attendant, guilt of non-performance, which all together keep a continuous tension rising.

6. The "pseudo-inflation" of minor annoyances: a diversion device to avoid major issues.

7. *Tension that immobilizes:* as in self-pity.

8. The tension of *worry* which lowers efficiency and diminishes action.

9. "Drop tension." On the way to apathy. When you take something in your hand and drop it, as if the nerve ends had made no contact with the object.

10. Tension wires that bind the breathing apparatus.

11. Bastion of Little Fears built into the body.

12. Habit Tensions.

13. Tensions caused by postural misalignment.

14. *Stifling the Process of Clarification.* Clients who repress insight and honest confrontation have been known to stiffen their bodies in a total way or to cramp it in parts.

This block of encrustation of tension results from the refusal to admit to psychophysical pain.

YOUR TENSION IS TAILORED BY OTHERS AND BY YOU TO SUIT INDIVIDUAL NEUROSIS.

Part Two, on Relaxation, will appear in an upcoming issue of *Sedona Life*.

Source SEDONA LIFE, Vol. III, No. 5, Sedona, Arizona 1978

Relaxation and Resilience
by Blanche Evan

Part One of this presentation, "Jagged Tensions and the Flow of Dance/Movement Therapy" appeared in Sedona Life, *Vol. III, No 5. In that article, Ms, Evan discussed tension and it various physical and psychological factors.*

In this article, Ms. Evan focuses her therapeutic techniques for the attainment of relaxation, and how steps can be taken by the "normal neurotic" to realize this desirable state.

For more information concerning Dance/Movement Therapy, please refer to Blanche's earlier articles in Vol. III, Nos. 2, 3, and 5 of Sedona Life Magazine.

PART TWO OF TWO PARTS

Life flow is Blood flow. Blood carries nutrients and vital gasses to every millimeter of the body. When this flow stops, the body dies - quickly and in minutes. And as we know, but take for granted, oxygen is decisive. Its integration with blood circulation sustains life.

What has this to do with relaxation? The fact is that tension produces over-contracted muscles which stop circulation, preventing the blood from gathering toxins and carrying them out of the body; whereas chemical equilibrium creates clear passage for *renewal of action*. This balance provides a base for resilience in psycho-physical behavior.

Physically, resilience connotes a state of reciprocal contraction and expendability of muscles (see Vol. III, No. 5, *Sedona Life*), thereby aiding rhythmic control of movement and its qualities. Resilience makes possible diverse qualities and freedoms of movement: legato smoothness, staccato clarity. Joints of the feet alive, knees yielding, torso upheld, spine verticalized and pliable, pelvis mobile, neck seeking to look *at* and *where*, arms vital, hands ready, and senses alert...

Psychologically, resilience is a state of readiness: body, mind and feeling merged for action, a state which fosters spontaneity and the immediacy for needed change. In summary, this is the opposite of what the neurotic client terms as "being stuck". Resilience, rare in these days, is always a challenge to deep-set resistance, to the flow of life and death and to the embrace of hate with love.

In our world, tension seems much more "natural" than relaxation. We should be able to go to a school to learn how to regulate our tensions, but such would be a difficult school to find. By contrast. there are dozens of workshops, methods, institutions, cults (materialistic, eclectic and mystical) that are mushrooming in this country, spoon-feeding relaxation of a dark color to their clients, mostly in forms of passive retreat. But why pass out into inertia; why blank out? To take your mind off what bothers you until next time it bothers you is a way of perpetuating what bothers you. It is time deferred. What way do you choose to "become calm" - to suppress your tension by *not* coping with it, or to quiet down, to change your body, and enlarge your insight?

As a practicing Dance/Movement/Word therapist, I treat tension and relaxation on a psycho-physical level with a physiologic approach to each individual's habitual mechanisms. This is directly opposed to ways and means that divert the human being *away* from self, leading him to oblivion, to psychedelic blow-up, and in the extreme, to submission to murderous and suicidal cultists and their ilk.

Simply stated, relaxation is a condition of *'let go'*; tension is a state of *'don't let go'*. Let go and let the blood flow. When you don't let go, *nerves* as well as muscles are involved, often coupled with as mind that tenaciously grips its negative memories to prolong pain. In *'let go'*, the spirit refuses to become the victim of tension. It is valid to say that an individual's tense or relaxed state is not only what "happens" to a person, but it is also what the individual does with "it".

Neurotic...Neurons...Nerves...Tension...Muscles...Contraction...*Neurosis*...

The best reference that I can suggest to clarify the relations among these areas is *PROGRESSIVE RELAXATION* by Edmund Jacobson, published in 1929, in which the author refers to the tonus of neuro-muscularity and to the relationship between the nervous system and the mind. The body and the mind are integrated; neither one is exclusive of the other. Fifty years later, in 1979, a large segment of therapy has not yet caught up with this concept.

Relaxed, but not apathetic. From Blanche Evan's film, *Retrospective*. Photo by P. Clagnez.

In a super-tense person, many muscles are contracting for no use whatsoever. *The nerves have taken over!* In the neurotic individual, the nerves dominate the scene. When the mind is filled with material that provokes tension, the neuro-muscular systems are affected. Some of the characteristics of the relaxed and resilient individual: not neurotic - conscious coordination of mind, body, thought and feeling; acceptance of the lift and drop of mood shared by all mammals, including mankind; common sense; self respect; wisdom to let go, with its ineffable rewards; power for action; growing up; acknowledging one's personality, one's potential and one's limitations. Letting go as a human being according to your psychophysical need in the place and time appropriate for you, which includes the different settings and levels of your way of life. These are all major ingredients in your tension-relaxation confrontation. You can take action, for example, in these areas:

FEARS

Some fears are valid. But reconsider them. Do you need them all? Are they of a specific nature or of a more general anxiety? Are they phobias?

Of course, fears cause tension of different kinds. Many clients I have worked with equate tension with power - and are *afraid* of losing power or control even momentarily in their work or in their sexuality. Now turn around; activate your mind *toward* your body rather than inward to your mind. Visualize a tension-apathy map of your own body. If you don't know how to draw, basic skeletal, muscular and circulatory maps are easily available. Identify your over-contracted muscles and apathetic drift. Seperate the knots; consider releasing the contractures that have resulted from *habitual* strain. Ask yourself: where and when are you rigid? In social situations, in intimate contact, in school, in work? Examine your 24-hour day; slow down and cut down on at least the more obvious self-destructive actions and reactions.

INITIAL SUGGESTIONS:

Body mechanics: if you have to hold, lift or carry a heavy weight, don't tense your knees; let them help you by giving, by bending. Do not use effort and strain. Stay within the bounds of what the task requires.

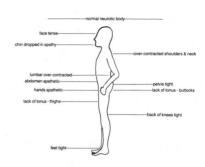

By contrast, if you are excessively dropping things, then concentrate on the object and grasp it with more purpose, using more muscular contractions in the grasp. Heighten the input into the body, into the task.

Hydrotherapy: water as a medium. If you are apathetic, take a shower or go for a swim to increase *circulation*. At home, dilute Epsom salts and sea salt in a warm tub to soak out your exhaustion. It really works.

And so does *massage*--the old fashioned kind. Just massage to reduce fatigue from toxin retention.

Sleep: When you go to bed, use pillows under your neck, under the lumbar area of the spine, and around any joints that seem sore, like knees or elbows. And if you are afraid of the dark, leave a night light on instead of being "brave", without any light.

YOUR RIGHT TO BE

If your "visiting" obligations result in tension, then try to limit their time span. In other words, give your self *the right of your own time*. If you are always tired, investigate the cause; it could be anemia, insufficient nutrition, bad posture, or even bad shoes. Perhaps you feel proud of being tired, that you're at least not guilty of slacking. See your time schedules as more flexible and rearrange them. Perhaps someone or something *can wait*. Or don't *you* count?

Move: Nature made the human being to move; therefore, anyone can dance. Play a drum recording or something else with a beat, and dance. Abandoned loose-jointed movement may not be conventionally restful, but it is certainly an effective way to relax--if you can enjoy it. To *try* to relax by any method makes one more tense, and to dance freely is a way of relaxing by *not* resting.

Speak, Hum, Sing: Listen to your own voice. Can you hear it? Is it screechy? Are you muffing or straining your vocal cords? You don't have to scream or yell, symbolically or realistically, to be heard. But you do have to be heard in this culture of constant sound and noise that drowns out the human voice. People in America are on the move, wondering where to find peace and quiet, both in one's self and in the environment (Not everyone can live in Sedona). How and where can one be relaxed without making a fuss about it, without relying on one system or another to maintain it? If you can't get out of the city, then at least learn how to keep yourself from being destroyed by *it*? Release your tension along the way so that it doesn't become a fixed neuro-muscular state. Become conscious and learn how to balance out the functional mechanisms with your expressive needs. If this all sounds like a do-it-yourself package, it is only the beginning. Seek *therapy* for the deep hidden causes and seek professional rehabilitation for the body. Aim toward a reintegration of body, mind, feelings and spirit.

Deal with the jagged lightning, seek out the flow of water and let it inundate your inner self - hear the raucous yelling, but learn to sing your own melody. Let it reverberate and let it be heard.

JAGGED LIGHTNING

Tension, sharp strikes...

Sudden bursts...

That sometimes frighten...

Staccato...

THE FLOW OF EASY WATER

Relaxation...

Soothing...

Allowing for continuum...

Enveloping relaxation...

Legato...

THE GOLDEN GATE

Resilience...

Give and Take...

Intensity and Quiet...

Dimension and Peace...

Openness to Action...

Functional Receptivity...

Renewal...

Source: <u>Sedona Life</u>, Vol. IV, No. 1 Sedona, Arizona, 1979

Articles About and Interviews With Blanche Evan

1941 — 1982

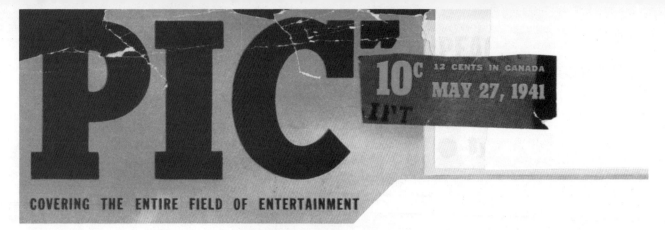

COVERING THE ENTIRE FIELD OF ENTERTAINMENT

TERPSICUTIES

THE child is a miniature volcano bursting with wonder at the world in which he has been placed, but--because he is not properly encouraged to give vent to his feelings--seldom do his creative potentialities "erupt." Such is the philosophy of Blanche Evan, New York dancing teacher. In the seven years that she has had children under her supervision, Miss Evan has operated on the theory that the dancing teacher must place no more emphasis on dancing *per se* than on the physical, emotional, and intellectual development of every child entrusted to her. To achieve this purpose, Miss Evan acts only as a "passive ally" in bringing out the youngsters' ideas. She *suggests* but never *commands*. And her students--which include boys and girls of four years and over from every walk of life--are so enthusiastic about the classes that even the most optimistic parents are amazed at the rapid and effective results. When a shy child comes into the class with a pronounced "I want to be alone" complex, Miss Evan calls out the percussion instruments (tom-toms, cymbals, gongs, drums), and the room is made so conducive to expression that the most backward child loses his self-consciousness almost immediately. In like manner, the boy or girl with an overbearing personality is placed in situations which prompt humility; again the results are like magic, and the most domineering child becomes "one of the gang" in jig-time.

Although the children use a great deal of energy in their many forms of play, the development of numerous muscles is neglected; thus the stomach remains soft, the arch of the foot weak, the shoulders round, the chest sunken. To make corrective exercises attractive to her students, Miss Evan offers a variety of pleasant calisthenics. In the "technique-images" method, the up-and-down flexure of the ankle is presented to the youngsters as a "see-saw ride for an ant"; lying on the back to lift the chest becomes "raising and lowering the Queensboro Bridge"; lifting the legs in circular rotation is "giving Suzie a ride on a ferris wheel--and you must keep your knees straight if you don't want her to fall out!" The second technique group concerns itself with movement principles, again built around the child's activity and imagination. For example, to encourage (a) speed, the youngster is asked to imitate a bird flying (running with co-ordinated arm action) to protect its little ones from an impending storm; (b) elevation--a frog jumping on the grass (frogs *never* land with a thud!); (c) balance--a butterfly pauses on the petal of a fragile flower. These are only a few of the techniques employed by Miss Evan to recondition the child's body, stimulate his imagination, and develop his personality, but they give some idea as to Miss Evan's teaching psychology. The accompanying photographs, made exclusively for "PIC" by Roland Harvey, show Minda Ware and Cecile Berkenfeld "at work" during a regular class.

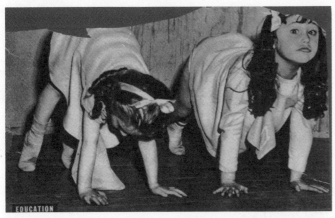

Building a bridge—which is big and heavy and must go up very slowly!—is good exercise for the legs, arms, back, and neck.

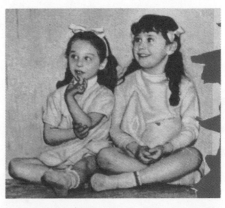

TIME-OUT PERIOD. Miss Evan, always careful not to over-exert her little pupils, divides the lessons in such a way that pauses like this one are rarely necessary. Individual class members tell stories during the recesses.

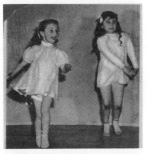

Showing how to swing and sway gracefully.

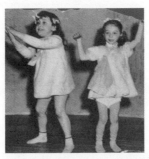

"Chopping Wood: strengthens little shoulders.

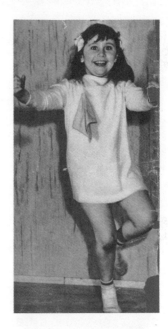

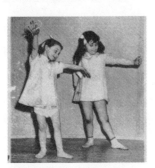

Movement exercise — Minda doing the creating.

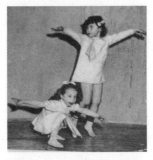

"Duck Walk" is recommended by football coaches.

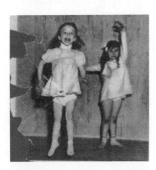

Light Landings come easy to the children when they make believe that it is Winter and they are jumping into a snowdrift. Hard landing would spoil the illusion.

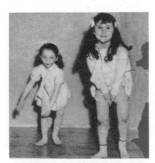

Imitations Produced by the little girls themselves are not always easily interpreted by adult observers, but they give the children confidence in thier creative ability and are body-cuilders.

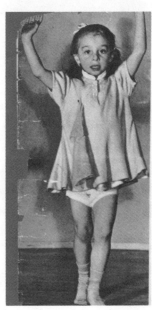

SEPTEMBER 1945 25¢   ON REARING CHILDREN FROM CRIB TO COLLEGE

PARENTS'

With Special Sections on
THE FAMILY HOME
FEEDING THE FAMILY
FAMILY FASHIONS
FAMILY FUN
735,000 Paid Circulation

MAGAZINE

Self-Expression Is A *Safety Valve*

By *Blanche Evan*

Director, School of Dance Development

Dancing and the other arts give young people a needed outlet for their loves and hates, their hopes and fears and frustrations

FOR THE ADOLESCENT, the period from eleven to fourteen is a kind of no man's land. It is a time when body and mind and personality are undergoing changes that make the young person seem unlike his former self. His relation to the adults about him is new and different. Even those whom he had learned to take for granted and feel close to--especially his parents--may seem remote and nonunderstanding at this time of rapid growth and change.

Frequently adolescents rebel against many conventions. Sometimes they are iconoclastic in regard to religion. At times they may appear arrogant and sophisticated although more often than not they are actually fearful and confused concerning the facts of life. The girl may suddenly become cosmetic conscious, perhaps "boy crazy." If her desire for male companionship has no outlet, she may find sublimation in the voice of a Frank Sinatra since our society as yet does not provide for enough healthful coactivities for boys and girls in their early teens. Similarly, a boy who finds no normal and happy outlet for his developing self may get into difficulties and feel himself generally a misfit.

In my work with young people, I have had the advantage of watching a number of them develop from the eight-year-old stage to that of eleven to thirteen years; and I have found that qualities manifested in an eight-year-old continue through the adolescent stage and seem to indicate a "personality pattern." Iris, for instance, at the age of eight, created a dance full of mystery and hidden powers. Iris, at the age of eleven, creates a dance of hypnotism, still mysterious, still dealing with suppressed powers within herself, now finding an outlet by directing others to her will.

Of course, each year brings new changes. Eleven is different from twelve; and thirteen, the first "teen" year, sometimes marks a distinct turning point. Nevertheless, I think we can consider the years from eight to sixteen one long dynamic crescendo in which the child seems to hold on to the self she has been, while at the same time coping with the new forces she is meeting in life.

The relation between the adolescent and the home is at this time, as at all ages, of the utmost importance. The happiness of the boy or girl may well depend upon sympathy, understanding, and love, and upon that freedom at home which encourages frank discussions. If these are lacking, no substitute can be found. A boy or girl who does not feel at home in his adolescent years is likely to carry the scar for many years, and subconsciously forever.

Even when the home is all that is should be, the creative arts have an important part to play in adolescence. Very often the boy and girl find in their cultural pursuits their only creative outlet for a deep, coursing emotional life, and for those inhibitions secret even from themselves, and certainly secret from the world. In cases where the boy or girl, for any number of reasons, goes through a period of estrangement from parents, some form of creative expression can supply much-needed outlets for their emotions and can offer opportunities for expressing the young person's changing views.

The relation between teacher and parent is another factor of great importance in dealing with adolescent problems. Ideally, there would be such rapport between teacher and parents of adolescent pupils as to make exchange of knowledge a natural procedure. And I mean more than the cursory question usually asked: "How is my child doing?" and the equally cursory reply: "Getting along well." I mean an analysis of the personality of the boy or girl, a knowledge of the home background and of behavior in other activities. I mean a discussion and an analysis of what the young person has unconsciously revealed in creative work, so that this knowledge might be consciously and constructively used by both parent and teacher to better understand the student and to assist him. Such a procedure carries creative art beyond the values of self-expression itself.

In order to gain such understanding, parents would have to be aware, in addition to the physical and educational needs of their children, of their emotional needs as well. Adults have been too prone to smile away the common complaint of the adolescent: "No one understands me."

Also, parents would have to become more objective concerning their own relations to their children, and more shockproof. In regard to art activities, they would have to recognize wider objectives than mere skill. They would have to realize that although the art teacher may see the student for only an hour or so a week the activity is such a concentrated one, that the teacher can learn much in this time about the girl or boy.

Perhaps I am putting the cart before the horse. Perhaps the first need is for more teachers in the arts to become conscious of the tremendous responsibility which is theirs in working with children of any age. There is still too little awareness that creative expression can be an important revelation of the student and should be used to further the development of his whole being.

In my own field, that of the dance, in addition to the technical work, I spend part of each lesson time on creative improvisations in which the pupils are encouraged to make up dances. The girls may come for lessons for any number of reasons: for better figures, better posture, grace, relaxation and so forth. However, through this creative outlet, a job of psychological house cleaning is often done which is invaluable to them. The students are never forced to explain their improvisations; but because an atmosphere of confidence in their teacher has been established, and an ever-growing self-confidence in the student has been nurtured, the girls are eager to explain their dances, although they are completely naively unaware of the revealing nature of their explanations.

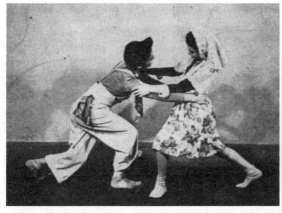 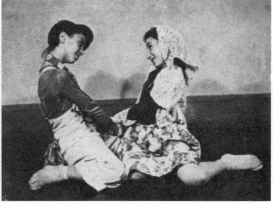

In their dancing class improvisations the adolescents' thoughts most often turn to love

"MY DANCE I want to be about living which is the slow walking and finding out about moving. Gradually I find I can do things with my body and dance freely!"

More succinct than any words an adult might choose, these sentences written by an adolescent in the dance class express the desires, point to the motivations, and indicate the psychological problems of many adolescents. We say glibly "She's all arms and legs...so awkward...He's so gawky...so unattractive..." These describe only the physical aspects of adolescence, and like many generalizations which eventually outwear their truth, no longer typify the boys and girls between the ages of eleven and fourteen, many of whom are not awkward, not ungainly, and certainly not unattractive.

On the other hand, you will not find an adolescent who is not tentative in his approach to what are still to him the mysteries of life. He has passed the limitless curiosity of childhood, he is beginning to find out, sometimes healthfully, sometimes in a surreptitious manner about the relations of men and women, and yet has not attained the liberties of young adulthood. He is "between walls..." a description one of my pupils gave of one of her improvisations. The rest of her phrase was "...and I couldn't get out." This is most significant. Not only does the adolescent feel, in the words of another student "tied to something, like a ghost in a field," but, also, "I can't get away." The surprised parent might ask: "From what? I knew my child had her moods, but I never thought she actually felt such blockings."

These adolescents whom I quote are not unusual, and are, on the surface, happy young persons. Some of them have come from more liberal homes than others, some from sympathetic homes, others from homes less sympathetic; but all of them come from comfortable, economically secure homes. Yet underneath this comfortableness and surface happiness, lie frustrations, inhibitions, half-understood desires, and often an unhealthful relation to parents. Because so much lies beneath the surface only an educational approach which burrows beneath can get at these young people.

ONE adolescent offered the following improvisation in class. She pulled a chair to the center of the floor and in a rather elegant pose, sat absolutely still for the first two minutes of the music. That is a long time to restrain oneself from dancing to exciting music. Suddenly she got up and danced with exquisite abandon for another two minutes. As suddenly as she had left her chair, so precisely did she cut her dance at a climactic point, and return to her first quiescent position.

Although very curious, I casually inquired what her dance meant. "Well, you see," she said eagerly, "in the first part, my mother is in the room, and so I don't move. Then she leaves, and I quickly get up and dance. Then she comes back, so I stop." This girl comes from a home that gives her every educational opportunity, a home that presents an outward appearance of harmony. The mother is distressed because, as she says, her daughter is "moody," but she seems unaware that she is a factor in the girl's instability. Without such awareness, she cannot help her daughter with her problems of adolescence, even though she wants to.

If any case bears out the valuable role a teacher can play as a discoverer and as go-between, it is this one just cited, for the girl herself is not consciously aware of the frustration she feels in regard to her mother. She is happily acquiescent to her mother's wishes, even though these run counter to hers. For instance, the mother wants her daughter to study ballet, but the girl wants to study creative dance, preferring it to ballet. And yet, ask the girl how she feels about this or anything else and her only answer is, "I don't know--ask mother. It's up to her." It is interesting, too, that the mother warned the teacher that her daughter was lazy. It had never occurred to the mother that the reason for this might very well be that the girl had had too little opportunity to make her own decisions. Her daughter's work proved in countless ways that she was competent and willing, but in need of freedom to express her ideas and feelings, and a chance for cooperative activities.

In this particular case, the mother asked for a consultation. I told her what I had observed about her daughter, she gave me a picture of the girl at home, and we both felt at the end of the interview that a better adjustment had been made possible for the girl--and for her mother too--because of the enlightening information we had to offer each other.

Another mother came to me distressed because her daughter was unsocial, a talented musician, yet too frightened to perform for others, awkward physically, and most self-conscious. In the dance class, the girl found it difficult to improvise dances of her own; but finally, the theme that broke down her resistance to free creative work was that in which she represented the force of evil, killing everyone and everything in her path. Once she discovered this theme she never tired of dancing it out. And a revealing dance it was for this gentle, high-strung, retiring girl. Later on, through discussion in class which led to improvisations, we were able to find a constructive balance in the themes of good and evil, again proving the value of drawing to the surface what often lies deep buried. This girl's mother told me very naively that she constantly nagged her daughter: nagged her to stand in good posture, nagged her to practice, to play for people, to dance at parties. She was, apparently, never happy or satisfied with her child.

THE adolescent period is a difficult time for mothers as well as for boys and girls. Parents are tired and inclined to feel that they should be able to relax after years of conscientious care of young children. On the other hand, they begin to worry about their boy's or girl's future and often try too hard to give them all the opportunities they feel they should have. Very often, too, there is the disappointment of finding that their children do not seem to value the advantages they are offered, and do not agree with their parents as to the professions they should follow. Upset and worried, faced with their own adjustment to middle age, parents are apt to forget that their children are going through a difficult transitory stage.

Many adolescents feel uncertain, unloved. They crave a demonstrative love: the kind they had from their mothers in childhood, even though they may assume an attitude that seems to ward off any such expression of love.

The teacher who keeps her ears open--not out of curiosity, but to learn about her students--and who encourages free conversation, will hear week after week, remarks of which two are the most frequent: "Nobody loves me any more," and "If I don't practice the piano every day, or stand up straight, or what not--my mother keeps telling me I won't be popular and no one will want to marry me."

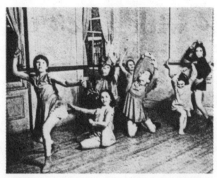
The girls are usually eager to explain their dances

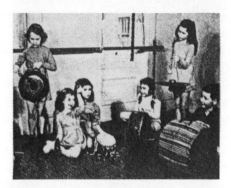
Children begin young to show their personality patterns

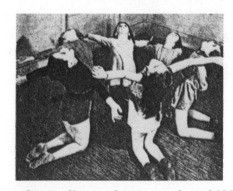
An understanding teacher can evaluate hidden meanings

Mothers often burden the adolescent with such standards and values that are not based on real values in education, that have no relation to joy, or taste, or the particular personality needs of the girl, but are based rather on the conventional standards of society. When, in addition, as often happens, the mother relates accomplishment to a competitive idea of marriage, the girl doesn't quite know what to make of it. She can't reconcile it with her burgeoning feelings of life and her need for love, love for parents and future mate alike.

A GIRL in one of my classes described the dance she composed as follows: "I was lonely. Then a man came. I was happy. He went away. I was sad. But he came back!" "And then?" "I was happy forever after!" Another girl asked week after week: "May we dance about the lovers?" In their improvisations, their thoughts most often turn to love. There are triangle situations--competition; there is the sure-of-herself girl with free choice. There is the evidence of fatalistic destiny: mystical love themes when sometimes the beloved dies. There are the girls who are aggressive and go after their suitors; the girls who are recessive and achieve their happy ending through a kind of dreamy wish fulfillment; and there are those who are dominating and get their lovers by hook or by crook or by hypnotism. There is sometimes the third figure, the mother, who prevents the girl from achieving happiness. Sometimes the mother intruder is won over, sometimes she is forced to accept the decision of the lovers. The ending is not always happy, but is sometimes tinged with great sorrow, even murder and death.

These themes are recurrent. Although they always appear to be spontaneous, they reach deep down into the adolescent kiln of living, of loving, and of groping. Adolescents should be given an opportunity to express the themes of their choice not only in dancing, but in all creative art forms--painting, poetry, dramatics and sculpture. Think what great therapeutic values lie in such expression. Think of the wisdom in providing creative outlets for what otherwise might well breed deep-seated frustration, cynicism, and distortion. And what valuable material there is in what the girl or boy unconsciously reveals. It can be used by teacher and parent, for the better understanding of the boy and girl. Since art study is capable of assuming such an interpretive role, what a loss it is to study the arts purely from the angle of acquiring techniques, with no thought given to the relation of the art to the forces that go to make up the inner life and being of the student.

Very often I have found in this age group, a mother, in her eagerness to give her child a well-rounded opportunity for education and accomplishment, allows the child to drift from one art study to another. When a change is made to meet the education or psychological needs of the young person, there is wisdom in it. When it is made in the spirit of dilettantism, the student and teacher are deprived of the necessary time for development, possible only through continued contact and work. The rate of gain in a second season is apt to be ten times rather than merely double. It is more advantageous to be a student of any one of the arts for several seasons than to get a smattering of different ones each year. The adolescent years are the time for the boy or girl to study the basic techniques of whatever form of artistic or creative work he wishes to do. Only in this way can the young person acquire a feeling of competence in his art work and a consciousness of the necessity for artistic discipline.

I find that the young person in this growing-up-fast stage is equally operative both in the creative work and in the technical phases of the work. He is usually eager to do the thing right and to do it thoroughly. If you--teacher and parent--understand the physical and psychological changes through which boys and girls go at this age and are willing to cope with phases of dreaming, spurts of temper, shyness, or the desire to dominate--if, in other words, you create the feeling that you are a real friend--you have an excellent chance of helping to turn darkness into the bright and happy future every adolescent wants so much.

Child Can Work off Urge For Violence In 'Free Expression' Creative Dancing.

By Dorothy Roe
AP Newsfeatures Writer

REPRINT — JULY 12, 1959

This is the somewhat simplified theory of Blanche Evan, who has been teaching creative dancing in New York City for the last 20 years, and finds that today's children have more violent feelings than ever before. Says she:

"Today's young people are constantly exposed to violence–in television comic books and movies. It's all around them all the time, and they are overstimulated by it.

"It's a difficult age altogether, for the young. They hear talk of atomic wars, of fantastic power, of voyages through space–and often one small child feels he's just not big enough to cope with all this."

Most of Miss Evan's dance pupils are girls--but there is no difference in their feelings of violence, and their need to express them.

"I find that the nice, well-brought-up girls from good families who come to my classes have tremendous repressions," she observes. "These are children of average families--the polite girls of our society. At first they resist free expression, but later they love it."

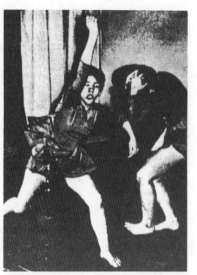

Lois and Leona both 13, students of Blanche Evan, let off steam in violent but harmless interpretive dance.

Miss Evan has found through the years that both small children and teen-agers find great joy and satisfaction in violent dances, which depict everything from fist-fights to murder. The modes of expression vary somewhat with the age. For instance, the 3-year-old likes to pretend to be an animal--a big wooly bear or a cuddly little kitten. From ages 6 to 9 children are preoccupied with speed--any kind of dance, just so its fast. From 10 to 12 they like to depict monsters, and in their teens are likely to express fears and uncertainty, which can be dispelled by violent action.

The dance as taught by Miss Evan has a great deal of psychology in it, and a number of her adult students are sent to her by psychotherapists.

"Psychiatrists are discovering more and more that bodily action can be an outlet for mental repressions," says Miss Evan. "My active body is necessary for a healthy mind. And our modern culture has put too much stress on intellectual achievements, too little on bodily activity."

After a dance session in which girls act out movements of violent anger and rhythmic mayhem, their teacher usually winds up the session with a quiet, peaceful dance about love or compassion.

"After they have worked *off* their feelings of violence they are ready for feelings of beauty and affection," explains Miss Evan. "to be able to love you also must be able to hate."

Miss Evan recalls an instance when a group of girls in the preteen age bracket were engaged in a dance in which they improvised motions of beating and killing. When the music stopped one gentle little girl was disappointed, saying:

"But I still had three more people to kill!"

These are normal, healthy expressions, says Miss Evan. And if children can let off steam in the imageries and actions of the dance, they're likely to be better adjusted to the strains of everyday life.

The Villager
Greenwich Village, New York

Thursday, June 12, 1969

She Made the Sun Come Out
For Her Many Young Pupils
by Morris Robert Morrison

One of those most prominently identified with the vanguard which first recognized the potential contribution of creative dance to the field of mental hygiene is BLANCHE EVAN, director of the Dance Therapy Center, 5 W. 20th St.

Nationally known for her series of articles in "Dance" magazine, subsequently reprinted as "The Child's World: Its Relation to Dance Pedagogy," she was the first dancer ever accepted for training at the Alfred Adler Institute of Individual Psychology.

Subsequently Miss Evan introduced the principles of dance therapy in a treatment program at the Children's Psychiatric Ward at Bellevue Hospital. After studying her work, Dr. Lawton in the first edition of "Dance Encyclopedia" in 1949, prophesied that "there is a whole new profession to be born...the profession of Dance Therapy."

Recently published figures indicate that the numbers of technicians trained in conventional psychiatry and clinical psychology grow proportionally fewer in their ratio to the accelerating incidence of emotional illness. Psychotherapists have begun to turn to such adjunctive aids as are inherent in the arts of music, painting, poetry and the dance.

More than 60 local psychiatrists and psychologists refer their clients to her classes where future therapists are also being trained. They have recognized a rare sincerity and dedication in her approach to the rehabilitative process as well as her unique and distinctive ability to handle children and adults in dance therapy work.

Miss Evan says, "In psycho-therapeutic practice there is considerable use for non-verbal communication. Cues to the patient's inner state can be deduced from body posture and movement. This can lead to an early confrontation which is difficult to secure in other ways. Diagnosis is followed by a course of treatment which aims to free the client of a sense of inferiority and self-consciousness. Energy formerly expended to maintain self-defeating attitudes is redirected towards exploring regenerating truths."

Creative dance which became a means of discovering and encounter with self first led to her present concentration on the therapeutic aspect of body awareness. At her center, which prepares future therapists, Miss Evan teaches her trainees to study the therapeutic effects of dance on themselves before assuming the responsibility of working with others.

While some purists shrink from the identification of art with therapy, Miss Evan, a leading theoretician in creative dance, whose bibliography in this area now numbers more than 50 titles maintains that the utilitarian and the aesthetic need not remain at odds. The aesthetic may indeed bring reinforcement to the purposeful. The issue is not whether beauty serves truth or truth beauty. In the final analysis, they are both one.

Many prominent theatrical personalities are former pupils of Miss Evan. They include Howard DiSilva, now starring as Benjamin Franklin in the hit musical, "1776." Speaking about him, Miss Evan said that as a student, "He performed the most fantastic improvisations I have ever seen in my life."

Michael Kidd, the famous dance and choreographer of Broadway and Hollywood's greatest musical shows, registered with her when she first gave a free course in dance to men. He stayed on for two years, abandoning a career in science for which he had been preparing as a chemistry major at college.

Other proteges include Renee Gluck, now an outstanding dancer in Israel, Marcia Kurtz who starred in "America Hurrah" and who has testified that "Blanche Evan changed my life," and Robert Theirkild, a principal in O'Horgan's "Tom Paine," who is presently in Hollywood preparing for a role in the movie version of "Futz."

"I Made the Sun Come Out." These are the words of a former pupil after the child had completed her own design for a new dance.

What Miss Evan hopes for her students is that they emerge from their concern for dance with a willingness to face the hazards of life and attempt to discover the inner reality of their experience. This, she feels means moving beyond catharsis--the letting out of feeling. Restoring wholesome and meaningful movement to the physical structure of the body also assists in refurbishing the psychic self.

She is in many ways an exemplar of her teaching.

Newsday
The Long Island Newspaper, N.Y.

10 Cents   Wednesday   Feb. 24, 1971

Behavior/II

Dance Therapy: A flourishing field
By Cheryl Bentsen

A crescendo of pounding drums fills the studio. Just before the pulsating rhythms become ear shattering, a young woman in a leotard places her drum aside, rises, and begins a gyrating dance. As the others watch, their beating subsides until the group sprawls on the floor in relaxation. This is a dance therapy session, and the dancers are all neurotic patients referred to BLANCHE EVAN'S Dance Therapy Centre in Manhattan.

Since 1946, when dance therapy was introduced to the mental health clinic of St. Elizabeth's Hospital in Washington, D.C., it has spread around the world helping psychotics, neurotics, the blind, retarded, and drug addicted; in hospitals and private studios. A number of universities now offer dance therapy courses, and several, following New York University's School of Education, plan to offer a master's degree in the field. An American Dance Therapy Association has been formed to devise standards to accredit therapists.

The techniques of dance therapy may run the gamut of psychological philosophies, but dance therapists all agree on the one general definition it was founded on: The integration of body and mind.

You can find MISS EVAN, the woman who started it all, perched on a stool in her studio most days observing her patients and occasionally jotting down notes on their movements. With the belief that "movement can't lie," as core of dance therapy, she can read their emotional problems through their posture. "Many patients conceal their unpleasant feelings behind a cheerful facade," she explained.

But once they're dancing, they give themselves away. For example the neurotic depressed patient will allow his body to sink down into gravity, his head and shoulders slouched. His back and pelvis are static, often indicating sexual frustration. During an improvisation about love his arms may droop emptily to his side, as if love were too painful to express. Movements will be small; and he may be afraid to move through space. The dead arms and rigid pelvis are key areas to Miss Evan's trained eye. The face, expressionless, is ultimately the last body area to be liberated.

For the psychotic patient, who, unlike the mere neurotic is often out of touch with reality, dance therapy can be a beginning. Lee Strauss, director of the dance therapy program at Bellevue Psychiatric Hospital said, "There are times when dance therapy is more useful than verbalization." Those sessions are voluntary and limited to twice a week due to a lack of funds, space and staff.

The techniques for psychotics are different from neurotics. Mrs. Strauss always plays music for psychotics; drums or nothing for neurotics. "Psychotic patients need the support of music because their defenses are up and their ego strength is minimal." Improvisations aren't used because they require use of the imagination that would detract from the pure, natural movements of the patients. "The very withdrawn will hardly move, maybe only his fingers, but it is something for him to just get his hands off his lap." The sessions help the patient get rid of lethargy as well as excess energy. For the neurotics, drums can "trigger" the liberation of the body from its inhibitions.

The patients often realize what their movements meant later after the therapy session. After an extremely aggressive session with severely regressed women, one of them asked to sit out the next session because she was tired. Later she told Mrs. Strauss she had been very contrary and agitated that morning, refusing to take her medicine. She was put in a separate room where, she explained, she began pounding and slamming the walls. But she told Mrs. Strauss that she had done this to calm herself and release her aggressive feelings, recalling how that kind of movement had helped her in the last therapy session. The women outnumber the men in Miss Evan's classes. "The false tradition of homosexuality in dance stops most men from coming," she said.

Miss Evan became interested in dance therapy long before there were teacher training courses such as the one she began in 1958. "My dance thinking has always been psychological," she said. "I always choreographed about people struggling in concentration camps, offices and slums, struggling to be themselves."

Her own dance training began when she played a lettuce leaf in a dance recital at age 7. After an extensive career as a dancer she became the first dancer to be accepted at the Alfred Adler Institute of Individual Psychology.

Free School
Boulder Colorado, 1978

'Normal Neurotics' Dance to Health
by Marda Kirn

Dance therapy has been brought out of the medical institutions and into the lives of "normal" people to help them resolve their emotional conflicts.

The re-emergence of dance as a therapeutic tool is the rediscovery of the body as the natural vehicle and outlet for the psyche, according to Blanche Evan, a world-famous dance therapist who will be leading a special Free School class this fall.

DANCE THERAPY WAS ORIGINALLY prescribed as a diagnostic tool in psychotherapy about 30 years ago. Used primarily with psychotics, the mentally retarded, and adults and children with perceptual and physical handicaps, dance therapy was effective in changing patients' outlooks on themselves and others.

As a dance therapist, Evan turned her attention from institutions to those who she calls "normal neurotics" those people who function normally but remain unfulfilled. From her observations of hundreds of children and adults in her school, she concluded that our social mores destroy physical spontaneity and today's mechanized life anesthesizes and "virtually immobilizes the body to minimum range." According to Evan, ninety percent of the population are normal neurotics, blocked by repressed emotions and fears with no hope of reaching their full creative potential.

Dance has been used in ceremonies and rituals for thousands of years, helping people to cope with anxieties and stress. This outlet was lost with the emergence of modern man and the subsequent decline of religious ceremony, particularly in Anglo Saxon countries.

THE ENGLISH LANGUAGE, according to Evan, has many examples of the symbolic acceptance of the role of the body as a natural, dynamic outlet of thought and action: "to face the challenge, to fly into a rage, to settle down, to stand up for your rights, etc."

Children use their bodies to express emotions. They kick their legs in screaming tantrums. They skip when joyful, curl up in laps when sad or insecure. But the transition to adulthood, children are taught to repress sexuality, anger, aggression and even sorrow in the name of "civilized" man.

Evan says, "In practical living, the body has been so severed from its role of expression that even the use of hand gesture is considered vulgar. Approved bodily expression is limited to games, sports and mechanical accessories where there is always a specific, and to all appearances, an impersonal objective." Although these activities are outlets for some emotions, those remaining suppressed are left to fester and can eventually become the seeds for neurosis.

Dance was further separated from daily life in the West by the development of ballet and modern dance, performed primarily in theatres by professionals highly trained in schools that emphasize technical virtuosity. Because of this, dance for most people became "something to see rather than to do." Today the notion that dance has to be a specialized, non-participatory art form is gradually changing as people feel less intimidated about trying it themselves.

AN INTRODUCTION DANCE THERAPY

For those who dance but who have not experienced dance therapy with Blanche Evan. Students will experience the differences between Creative Dance and depth exploration of self-movement as it evolves into the medium of dance/movement/word therapy. The basic indicator for the student client is the change from "Who am I?" to "What do I WANT to be?" along with the sorting our of Fantasy from Reality--to release bottled emotion, to make whole what is segmented, to activate potential.

For 20 years Blanche Evan has pioneered in dance therapy for that urban adult who functions yet remains unfulfilled. Blanche works privately in New York and Arizona : in universities in California and Boulder. She has originated her title: "Dance/Movement/Word Therapist", believing all three should be joined to effect successful therapy.

FOR MANY PEOPLE THE study of any form of dance has become a kind of therapy. But dance therapy is different. It is not, as commonly believed, a system of exercises designed to act as a panacea for faulty technique. The opposite of formal training, dance therapy "deals with the individual and his world rather than the history or skill of dance in its art and ethnic manifestations," says Evan. It "seeks to express rather than impress", dealing with not just the physical, but the psycho-physical, in an attempt to unify thought, feeling and body action.

Dance therapy is based on the "muscle memory" concept used by physical therapists. It states that the body has "automatic, involuntary response to emotional feelings." When emotions are repressed, this causes body tension, rigidity and non-productive movement patterns. Gestures and posture can reveal much about a person's underlying feelings of inferiority, self-consciousness, fears and frustrations which by words and social masks people hide from others and especially themselves. The dance therapist looks beyond these pretenses by diagnosing movements and directs the client through improvisational exercises designed to free him of self-defeating attitudes which block the actualization of human potential.

Through improvisation under the guidance of the dance therapist in the safe, controlled environment of the studio students "dance out" their emotions, releasing them from the body's muscular memory. Once feelings are exposed, students can become aware of and accept them for what they are--emotions. They can deal with them constructively by redirecting their insights toward change and personal growth.

Evan helps students further by prescribing corrective exercises based on functional technique to re-educate the muscles, to change the old and develop new movement habits, which re-enforce psycho-physical balance.

Ironically the benefits of dance therapy are usually obvious to everyone except the dancer. "Oh, all dance is therapy" is the response most often heard. But this response ignores the fact that dance therapy deals with the emotions. Evan has found that children and adults who have come to her with a professional background in either modern dance or ballet "have without exception found this foundation to be a stone wall barrier to creative work, to self-confidence in generating movement, and to dynamic, meaningful movement."

Daily Camera
Friday, May 23, 1980
Boulder, Colorado

Dance Therapist Changes Lives
By Vicki Groninger
For the Camera

Some people read music; BLANCHE EVAN reads bodies, especially moving bodies, with the finesse of a symphony conductor. She's been doing so for over 40 years, first as a dancer-choreographer in New York (she performed in Russia in the '30s), then as a pioneering teacher of creative dance for children and the founder of the Dancer Therapy Centre in New York in 1967. Having her in Boulder is like having Isadora Duncan in residence.

Miss Evan, who moved to Boulder in October, 1979, teaches creative dance classes and dance therapy workshops and sessions through the continuing education division at the University of Colorado, the Community Free School, and her own studio. Her work is for people who want to get back in touch with their bodies and their senses as the originators of their feelings, thoughts and behavior. To this end she applies dance as a primal therapy.

She switched her interest to helping those whom she calls "normal neurotics" after working with children for 20 years in New York City. As a result of this work, she published a classic series of articles, reprinted as "The Child's World," in Dance Magazine. She asked, "Since movement in the child is the natural vehicle and outlet for the psyche, why isn't this so for adults as well?" She observed that "the unification of body and emotion so natural in the child is destroyed in the process of growing up partially because our social mores repress physical spontaneity in adults but mostly because mechanical life has virtually immobilized the body to minimum range." She further described the syndrome: "To the private urban citizen (the 'normal neurotic'), to be civilized means to repress aggression and anger with no active alternative (such as physical work) supplied. Adrenalin, which is automatically produced in the body to cope with these feelings through action, has nowhere to go. With action repressed, the energy is diverted to different kinds of tension-- rigidity at one extreme and apathy at the other."

It is Evan's belief that Americans are searching with their customary inventiveness for movement that can release their pent-up feelings and unite the now-severed strains of body and mind. In Boulder especially, we pay a fortune in short-term installments to engage in the latest body therapy, healing art, mind trip, or sporting fanaticism for the peace of mind and sense of wholeness we hope to get.

But Evan thinks we are unlikely to achieve the satisfaction we are looking for in these ways. Furthermore, she believes that "thought stripped of expressive, individual action prolongs the time span of neurosis." In a wide-ranging interview she offered these insights:

Unlike many body/mind techniques which share some characteristics with dance therapy (breathing, posture, and sound, for instance), dance therapy works at getting at the causes for the clients' distress in the most primal, elementary way--self-directed movement. Evan says, "Creative dance breaks the crust. Dance therapy leads to unraveling the knots, to diagnosis, and to active life, brain, habit change. The education of the emotions (an Adlerian term) is also possible."

How does this get accomplished?

Blanche Evan's special perception as a dancer led her to study at the Alfred Adler Institute of Individual Psychology and the New School for Social Research in New York. The dances and films she choreographed explored assertiveness, aggression, pain and grief years before these became popular studies in psychology.

In the studio she doesn't waste time. She demands concentration, work and honesty of her students and clients. She relies on two primary means to get her people to uncover buried feelings and to enlighten themselves about their past behavior and their potential for change. These are the systems of Functional Technique and Improvisation.

Evan's functional technique is, in her words "corrective exercise designed to retrain muscles to move in relation to nature's design, in a rhythm of expansion and contraction." She says, "Spontaneity and resilience, two of the signposts of the well personality, are enhanced by the individual's discovery of his own rhythm and tempo." In functional technique classes she'll concentrate on movement in one body section at a time, often relating its working with its attached parts; if it's the arms and legs, with their related structures in the torso--the pelvis, buttocks, lumbar region, spine, rib cage, and complementary muscles. Each client finds his or her own range of movement, then works to increase it. As one of Evan's students in Boulder, Wanda Pishny of the Brent Mason ballet company, recapitulated, "Your muscles have memory. When they react without any conscious effort on your part to a given situation, they tell you where you are. By working to increase your range of movement, dance therapy purports to increase your range of coping and creative response."

But Evan's real genius is in improvisation. Paul Oertel of the Nancy Spanier dance company, like Spanier a longtime student of Evan's, says of her: "BLANCHE EVAN is brilliant. She sees behind people's masks and uses her own creative insight to set up experiences that will help her clients find their problem for themselves. She has a great ability to set up improvisations on her insights."

Evan defines improvisation as the spontaneous creation of form. Usually she will assign a these for student-clients to "dance out." In so doing, they are discouraged from trying to look pretty, moving from habit, judging themselves or feeling judged in any way. The movement may be to music, a drum-beat or silence. In private sessions, she dispenses with music because it can clutter the dancers' immersion in themselves. She says, "It provides an outside stimulus that evokes an aesthetic rather than psychophysically pure (individual, spontaneous) response."

Sometimes before a private or group session, Evan will have you write down a one-sentence statement of what you're feeling at the moment or what's bothering you. Then she'll have you choose an action word in your verbalization to dance or put into action. She says: "I have my people go from saying 'I feel' into doing that feeling, from saying 'I wish' into moving that fantasy."

Though she generally finds the hands and face to be the last defense outposts that each person will release, Evan thinks sound is where the normal neurotic is repressed--even more than in moving the face. She says, "Self-produced sounds seem to wake up the whole person in an immediate kind of way. The most difficult area is in production of throat and gut sounds related to the significance of the movement being expressed."

In response to dancing to themes, Blanche might "assign" in class, people often achieve a catharsis of their emotions. Expressing an emotion in movement, rather than just thinking it, has far-reaching ramifications in the individual's psychic life. It becomes much more real to you; you can't just wish it away once you've moved it; it's there in all its naked honesty to show you how you "really" feel. Then the mind takes over connecting this new expression of feeling with past sensations, remembrances. You begin to see a pattern of reaction in yourself and can then decide whether you like the pattern or want to change it.

In dance, unlike much other movement, the future can be acted out by using one's imagination. Today, Olympic runners talk about the role of visualization in their training. Boulder's Stan Mavis says, "I don't worry about the competition when I'm running past them. Before the race I've visualized myself running behind the pace car, so that's all I see until I get there."

One theory of dance therapy is that you can help bring about a better future for yourself by living in the present with the full force of your personality--your strengths--and coping with hopes, fears, and anxieties for the future a little in advance by dancing them out.

Evan says the dance therapist is uniquely prepared to help people confront their own experience directly, to break through their resistance to self-creativity. She equates this resistance with fear--the fear of making a statement, of risking being different from someone else--and with the peculiarly American propensity to split personality, separating feeling from thought, body from mind (sex from love, love from hate...) Also, dance therapy helps people develop confidence in their own identities and the strength to pursue those identities in spite of the destructive forces in society.

One of Evan's students in New York described the work as "actualizing energy which has been trapped and is working to hold in rather than let out feelings." Others who have participated in sessions Evan holds throughout the country have shown three prevalent reactions: You lose the illusion that there's anyone else in the world besides yourself who can take responsibility for who you are and what you do; you develop insight into the causes of how you turned out the way you are; and you begin to perceive what you can count on in yourself to better direct your life.

Evan sums up this basic aim of dance therapy: "If you find your strengths, you can begin to develop your own individuality. (Creative dance provides the atmosphere for non-conformity.) You ask yourself. 'What can I do to find satisfaction?' Finally, after a lot of work you have a 'you' to give to yourself and maybe to someone else and then perhaps you can begin to receive."

Because you've moved to get your insights they're more likely to have a greater impact on you than if they had just been spoken in verbal therapy.

Evan's work has been life-sustaining to herself in more ways than one. Recently, when she was giving a deposition in a court case, the opposing lawyer, astonished at her vitality, asked, "Have you found the fountain of youth?" Evan answered confidently, "Yes."

"Well, where is it?" he importuned. Rising to the fullness of her petite height, Evan answered, "It is the art of dance."

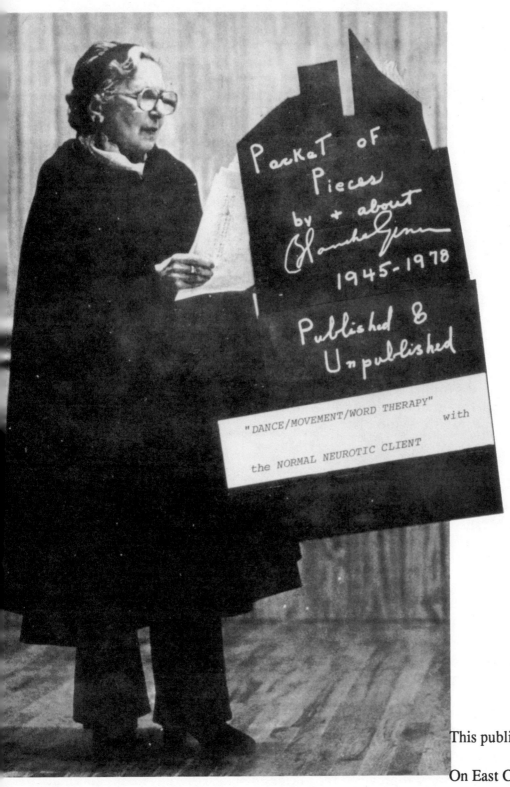

This publication available as follows:

On East Coast:
    Att: Barbara Melson
    129 Columbia Heights
    Brooklyn, NY 11201

On West Coast:
    Att: Anne Krantz
    146 Fifth Avenue
    San Francisco, CA 94118

AMERICAN JOURNAL OF DANCE THERAPY
Volume 5 — 1982

An Interview with Blanche Evan

Blanche Evan, DTR
Founder and Director, Dance Therapy Centre
Faculty, Alfred Adler Institute of Individual Psychology
Private Practice

Iris Rifkin-Gainer, DTR
Adjunct Assistant Professor
Department of Dance and Dance Education
Graduate Dance Therapy Program
New York University

Belief in the art of dance as creative transformation has permeated the work of Blanche Evan. She has pioneered in the fields of dance, choreography, dance teaching, and dance therapy for over 50 years. As recently as 1981, she was commissioned to choreograph a piece for California-based dancer Anne Krantz. In the same year, The Scholarship Project in Boulder, Colorado was privately funded for the summer of 1981 with the express stipulation that the work of Miss Evan become more widely known.

I have had the unique experience of a continuing relationship with Miss Evan since 1947. I attended the marvelous creative dance classes for children in which she specialized for over 20 years. Her unique and rich contribution in this area is documented in her book *The Child's World: It's Relation to Dance Pedagogy*, of which she recently said: "I really believe that anybody interested in my evolution as a dance therapist would get to know me and the work by reading *The Child's World*." In the late 50's, as I grew into adolescence, we were guided to dance out themes which expressed our inner conflicts and those of the family and world around us. This work was to develop into her approach to dance therapy.

In 1967 The Dance Therapy Centre in New York City, founded and directed by Blanche Evan, opened its doors. For the next nine years it provided the nucleus of dance therapy for the "normal neurotic urban adult." People came from many countries to train with Miss Evan, as well as from the United States. Despite her peripatetic life-style, I have been fortunate enough to study dance therapy with her periodically from the '70's to the present.

Miss Evan is currently active as a dance therapist and teacher throughout the United States. Over the years, she has presented her material in New York University's Department of Adult Education, the Graduate Dance Therapy Programs of both New York University and Hunter College, Evergreeen College in Olympia Washington, the University of Colorado in Boulder, and has given dance therapy workshops across the country. Dance therapists trained in her methods carry on her work in New York, San Francisco, Paris, Israel, and London.

Her prophetic article in *The American Dancer* (1938), in which Miss Evan foresaw the coming together of "opposite" forms of dance such as ballet and modern, is one of over 40 articles to appear in various periodicals including *Dance Magazine* and *Dance Observer*. Her published works include the aforementioned *The Child's World: It's Relation to Dance Pedagogy* and *Packet of Pieces--Dance / Movement / Word Therapy with the Normal Neurotic Client*. Within the year the first presentation of her system of "Functional Technique" will be published. In addition, three films of her work are filed in the Dance Film Archives of Lincoln Center.

In this interview, Miss Evan recalls her early influences, discusses her professional development, and states some current interests and passions in her work.

Iris:Blanche, is there anything in your early history that particularly contributed to your development as a dancer and dance therapist.

Blanche: One of my lovely childhood memories relates to Public School No. 17 (which is still on 47th Street in Manhattan, and to Mrs. August Belmont who was a philanthropist and who offered the children courses in drama and dance led by two beautiful ladies, Miss Ford, for drama, and Mrs. Simmons, for dance. I was seven or eight. The production was to be at the Century Theatre, which was a very, very large and beautiful, ancient theatre. Both teachers wanted me for a main part, a child's part, and I had to decide whether I wanted to dance or act in the play. I loved both teachers, but I loved dance more than anything it seems, even at that age, and I have never deviated.

I: And later,

Blanche: As a young adolescent, I studied ballet with Mme. Stavrova. I left after a while, and I found a teacher, Miss Bird Larson, who was teaching a form of dance--it was then alluded to as "rhythmic dancing"--that I felt was right for me. Her technique was derived from movement healthful for the body, yet open to skill. We never *imitated* "a form." Within two-and-a-half years I was placed in the advanced class. Bird Larson died suddenly. I felt myself an orphan.

I: Were you also performing at that time?

Blanche: My first authentic solo recital was in the Village. I was 18 1/2 years of age. Later, I gave solo performances in Boston, New York, and in West Virginia, with an orchestra. I performed in colleges: Hunter, McGill, and the North Carolina Negro College in Durham, and in Raleigh. I created dances of labor, of anti-fascism, and delicate dances with bells on my feet. I did a dance, a kind of emerging dance, which seemed to me to speak of some spiritual place. My last major work was "Death of the Loved One" (1946), for which I wrote the words and arranged the music. Doris Humphrey commended me on the choreography.

I: And when did you begin teaching?

Blanche: I believe I began teaching after the death of Bird Larson; she was only 40 when she died. And therein lies my fate. I taught friends, at first, adults. I remember that I still called my work rhythmic dancing. I don't know when I switched to creative dance. By the way, I don't like that title anymore either.

I: What would you prefer to call it?

Blanche: I don't know. But the more I'm involved with dance and dance therapy, as experience of one's totality, I feel that none of these titles really say what I mean in the way that I dance and in the way that I teach dance and conduct dance therapy. I never called myself a modern dancer.

I: What would you say was the next step, or the next branching out, in you career?

Blanche: I had done my first professional job of teaching and performing in Montreal, in the year 1931-32, and when that was finished, I wanted to catch up with my studies again in New York. I did an intensive course with Martha Graham, a full season with Hanya Holm and Louise Kloepper, a course with Louis Horst, and a choreography course with Doris Humphrey. *New Theatre Magazine, New Masses,* and *Theatre Arts Monthly* published my articles which responded to the modern dance of that time; also my piece on the legacy of Nijinsky and Duncan. From that point on I was isolated in the field. After the clear viewpoint of Larson I couldn't identify with the major schools. This isolation was very serious.

When I came back to New York from Montreal, I was with the Roerich Museum and the Albertina Rasch Studio for two seasons. Then I opened my own studio in 1934 and continued for 40 years to have a New York studio, until 1975. I had worked mostly with adults. But when I opened my studio, children came; they seemed to come from nowhere, or from somewhere, because I never sought them out. For the next 20 years I was a specialist in creative dance for children.

After I had become a concert dancer, I resumed my study of ballet with Ella Daganova who was a wonderful teacher in the Cecchetti method, and then Vilzak-Sholler; also Spanish dance with Veola, who was Escundero's teacher; Indian and Hawaiian Dance with La Meri, and an unforgettable intensive with Harold Kreutzberg. I travelled to far places and saw folk and theatre dances of Spain and Portugal, a national folk dance evening in Kiev done by sailors, farmers, and other workers from all over the Soviet Union, and the Volador Flying Pole Dances in Paplanta, Mexico. I studied Haitian dance daily in Haiti for three months. I gave a concert in the Park of Culture and Rest in Moscow where the director presented me with a medal of appreciation. On the Island of Ibiza, at the end of a fiesta day, I was asked to do a spontaneous presentation for the island people.

In the studios I mentioned, many of my classmates were people who then became famous in the theatre and in dance: Jerome Robbins, Michael Kidd, Agnes de Mille, George Zoritch, etc. I was in Benjamin Zemach's Dance Company in the Max Reinhardt production *The Eternal Road* which ran for six months in New York, and sometime later in Elsa Findlay's *Orpheus*. Along the way I gathered experience appearing in smaller dance companies: Dhimah's Trio, Von Grona's and Jean Hamliton's Quartets. I even did one burlesque show with a partner who lost her wig. God, I could have killed her! That was really the end of any commercial ventures, although I did support myself dancing in art cafes.

During the war I was a volunteer dance teacher at Bellevue in the psychotic children's ward. I didn't yet know the name of Freud. Loretta Bender, head of the department, admired my reports on the patients in my classes and requested that I submit them for staff review. I remember in the dance class tracking down the secret of an 11 year old girl whose burden was her persistent incestuous father.

I: Can you say more on what you call your psychological bent?

Blanche: Yes. I never looked *at* anything, even as a child, but rather *through*. I seemed particularly drawn to the person who was struggling and who lacked the nourishment of basic elements in life. In much of my solo choreography the themes were of these people. In my "Slum Street Suite", one of the characters was the "Woman in Need." I went down to the East side of New York and looked. The women weren't bag ladies then, but they were ladies who dove into the trash cans, and I remember a very close friend making a trash basket for me that looked like those receptacles. At the end of the dance, I got into the wire basket and rolled around the stage in it. The accompaniment was a difficult piece by Prokofiev.

I had empathy and insight and association with these downtrodden women of reality. Certain dancers on their rise to fame, when they came backstage, said "Blanche, must you do dances like that?"

I: What were the elements that were responsible for the transition in your work from creative dance into dance therapy?

Blanche: The turning point was in the spring of 1958, in my New York demonstration: "The Psychological Content of Children's Creative Dance", in which children aged three through 18 participated. For the first time I felt I had the right to use the word "psychological" content. I had completed my own verbal therapy, and I had presented a paper "Life is Movement" to the Adler Center of Individual Psychology where I was a student. By 1958 children were changing from the wonderful creative child to the more materialistic kind of child who wanted *things* rather than feelings. Society at that time seemed to be going in one direction, and I was looking for another direction of my own. I knew then that I wanted to couple therapy with dance and to concentrate on adults. I had read that one out of 10 adults in America was hospitalized for mental disorders. I was most interested in the other nine. I saw a demonstration of Marion Chace's work at Turtle Bay Music School. Some of my own adult students were participating in that and I knew again that I preferred to work with the neurotic rather than the psychotic patient. I also took a course in abnormal psychology at the New School [for Social Research in New York City]. In September 1958 I offered my first course for dance teachers who thought they wanted to be dance therapists.

I: What are the most important elements to you and in you as a dance therapist?

Blanche: I think that the most important ingredient in me is what I've been talking about: to regard a human being, first of all, with respect...I remember this as true when I worked with little three year old children, the difference was in the life experience, the span of life. I never spoke *down* to a child and I never changed my voice into a little "itsy-bitsy-witsy for little little girls" because the child was perfect in her childhood and I had to find the bridge to the child and feel, through her, the limitations of her life as well as that great wonderment that children have. And I feel that with an adult it's very, very difficult because the adult is in trouble and I have to try and see through that trouble to find the person that was born many years ago, so we then have the possibility of working from the characteristics and strengths of the born self...in other words, it's *not* focus on *memory alone*, which is so much a part of therapy, but on *discovery*: what was the client born with that is endemic and cannot be erased anymore, endemic as the adult color of the eyes. The roots of a tree are deep and brown, invisible to the eye, yet it is they that are the source of nourishment. There is much hard work involved here, because the client herself has long forgotten her strengths and life has been difficult, and life *is* difficult, and very often a client is discouraged for a long time in therapy, the roots are so far back in her history. (I say "her" because most of my clients are female, and it is easier than saying her/his, etc.) To create continuity a client needs to carry out of the session something that she will work with until the next session.

I: How do you begin with a new client?

Blanche: I rarely give verbal interviews. Generally, I give the client a little piece of scrap paper which says on it: "Name dance experience. Name therapy experience. What is your age and your most difficult problem today?" And that's it. It leaves me open in the first encounter and helps to orient the client to her body as instrument rather than to her exclusive head.

When I speak of dance therapy I don't speak of "dance, semicolon, therapy, semicolon". My big objective and my fight in the field of dance therapy is the integration of dance *with* therapy, so that it becomes one. One, not that the dance is added to the therapy, but that it is "Dance: A Basic Therapy".

I: What about the client who's never danced?

Blanche: We wouldn't start with dance, but with the components of dance: with awareness of tension in its chronic forms and its use as repression; or with heartbeat or habit movement versus expressive dance; or with consciousness of movement habits. There are many ways. Sometimes a novice in this work, even in the very first session, creates a beautiful improvisation, beautiful because it derives from a desire *to do* and because it has touched her and she is beginning to contact some depth in herself; her unique self. Every self *is* unique.

Therapy is change. Therapy without change can be an endless walk in the desert. Good therapy results in change of attitudes and style of life and living; change in the body and changes in communication. Purification in advanced work is achieved when the client's quest for change becomes the unmitigated pursuit of change. The limitations of the therapist are co-existent with the limitations of the progress of the client.

I: It is unusual for a system of dance therapy to include a specific body technique, yet Functional Technique is an integral part of your work. Would you introduce us here to its fundamentals?

Blanche: Because nothing has been published on the subject, not many people in the field know of my method of Functional Technique. It is the system I created for building mobility, resiliency, unstylized skill, and strength related to personal structure. Living kinesis. It deals with bodily rehabilitation. And often that means dealing with structural defects or with the results of accidents of which the patient is often unaware. First of all, it is not taught to the client until she is well along in the work of dealing with her psychophysical problems and expressing them with her body whatever present state that body is in. The object is first *not* to change the body of the client but to let the client become freer and freer in exposing the body that she *has*. For instance, in the case of balance, the client needs to expose her fear of balancing or situations where she becomes unbalanced, to expose it and then to look at the body that is doing the distressing action and gradually to reach the point where she knows that if her body will change, her balance will change. At that point, functional technique will be introduced. It would include emphasis on the formation of the feet, the impacted rigidity of the knees, the recessive groin. The model is the norm. That is only part of the story of balance. Functional Technique is a technique of wide range.

I: Are there any other elements you would include here?

Blanche: Yes, intuition. In many training courses that I have given, I have rarely if ever felt that I could successfully teach the use of intuitive powers. The therapy is enhanced by insight--to cite inwardly. To go to the place where all this turbulence is going on, where all the depression is going on, and to draw out of that the elements that are connected with the client who doesn't even know that those elements are there. Because with her, they are buried in the unconscious; the task becomes how to lead her unconscious to consciousness so that the client can eventually face up to the mass of unconscious directives that she's living with, and by which she is abiding. These are psychophysical, not mental, and they serve her neurotic needs.

I: What about the current world she lives in?

Blanche: Very early in my work, I distinguished between social and personal neuroses, the latter going back to the family and early environment--and which in turn relate to the social neuroses of the parents. At some point in therapy the client has to, what I call, "let somebody in". If she doesn't open up eventually to include both the outside world and the intimate family world that she's obsessed with, therapy is at a standstill. She has to go out into the world and very often back, in a mature way befitting her age, to the parents.

In America, the ambition to succeed is paramount. The client has become competitive and mostly *self-competitive*, yet there is little clarity in life choices, including that of career. And, at 30 years, "should I have a baby?" "And if so, should I be a single parent?" And then, there's the city. Except for my wide travels, I've lived in New York all my life. I used to call New York the City of Stone, when I was really struggling to develop my work without the support of the city. Later I changed some of that stone into a plot where a tree could grow. Now I think of New York as the "Utmost City". If you really survive with some of the wonderful qualities nature has given us all, the City of Stone has not won.

I: What about the influences other than the city's on what you call the "typical American urban neurotic?"

Blanche: Well, I could quote from the clients who have said to me "my head is cut off from my body." And one said it beautifully: "When I came I felt I was a walking mind, and that has changed." One night in the therapy group, I said "every time you begin to what you call 'think' put your hand up." They were dancing away with their arms shooting up toward the ceiling, and finally they burst into laughter because they realized that most of what they were doing was listening to their heads go on and on--that wasn't even thinking. I really believe that good thinking includes feeling and good feeling includes thinking. Both are in the brain and in the body. The body is the overall containment. The body is everything that we are. Nature made the human body in terms of muscles, bones, joints, circulation, and nerves; a unique spinal verticality and a glandular seat of emotions; also sexuality, power of the brain, and character of will. Dance therapy can achieve reunion in the segmented self. The mind can become clarified, the feeling restored to vibrancy, and the client once again can claim her body as her own.

I: You don't see dance therapy as an adjunctive therapy?

Blanche: No. Absolutely not. When I became a therapist, in some cases, I was an adjunctive therapist. Rarely was there support from the verbal therapist. The more I worked with their referrals the more I realized I was doing work in my private studio which the therapist himself did not comprehend, though the client was greatly aided.

I: Through the years you have had a profound influence on many individuals, including myself, who have gone on to become dance therapists. In a new center for training therapists what would be some of your basic requirements?

Blanche: First of all, a person who wants to be a dance therapist for the neurotic client should have been trained in dance and she should have had exposure to therapy...

I: What other training is needed?

Blanche: Experience and training in my system of Functional Technique, my methods of improvisation, history of dance, dance therapy in other cultures, dance studies, choreography, and depth experience in personal dance therapy--all would be necessary. Also, sound in forms of percussion and music; space in terms of space content--and on and on. We also work on language. Just as the person enters the training with habit body movement and packed -in tensions and apathies which have lost their original reason for being, so this person uses language and verbal concepts without true relationship to therapy problems. In our work, language undergoes revision for the sake of specificity and selective use in dance therapy.

I: I remember much self-research, homework, and reading lists.

Blanche: I always give assignments to trainees which really get down to what you know, what you don't know, and what you need to know. Assignments are useful in amalgamation of all the issues that come up in dance therapy. There is also the matter of application of my work to different populations: to children as differentiated from the adult, to the normal neurotic child, to the disabled person, to the retarded, and to the elderly. In other words, dance therapy for the functioning neurotic does not exclude work with the above.

I: Is there anything that you haven't mentioned that you would include in that training?

Blanche: I'm sure there is--massage, nutrition, and aikido, for starters. And, especially in America today where many cultures are present and where they color a great deal of our lives in ways undetected before, the trainee must have an understanding of the client's social derivation and ethnic background. Training and self--this is the training program.

I: You have said the dance therapy trainee can't exist in an ivory tower.

Blanche: Yes!

I: How much time would be required to complete a training course in your methods?

Blanche: Three full years, five days a week, plus a year of supervised practice.

I: You spoke of language, and the word has permeated your work in various ways. In your professional evolution you have gone from naming your work "Dance," "Creative Dance," "Therapeutic Aspects of Creative Dance," and "Creative Dance in Therapy," to "Dance Therapy," and later to "Dance/Movement Therapy," and "Dance/ Movement/Word Therapy." Why do you include "word" at this point?

Blanche: I include it because I believe that the use of words in therapy is essential in our time. Everybody is talking in sessions. No therapy is valid in our society without the use of meaningful words. I know of no therapy in the arts that can dispense with the word. However, what kind of words are we talking about? Now this is a big part of our therapy. Vocabulary in our times always changes. I didn't know what a "punk" was until I saw the dyed hair in the street--and I think that's terrible, I should know. That is part of the world that the client has to deal with.

Everybody loves and yet the word "loves" seems to have lost meaning. Has love become a synonym for sex? Sex--the advertising, the legs turned upside down in a store that sells hosiery--I think a demeaning kind of attitude is prevalent in the commercialism that I abhor. And so, what does the word mean? "Sharing" is another word like that. Well I may as well tell you, we have a list of words that we're not allowed to use in my therapy, because of the lack of clarity to both the therapist and the client herself of what the client means. My intention is to cleanse the word of conventional use, since such use only perpetuates the blocks and defenses of the client. I find that clients use, when they don't know what else to say, "I have to get centered". I don't believe that Isadora used the word "centered"--and she seems to have found a place in her body where she could go as a source of quiet and concentration. She used it; as an emotional source, not as a label.

Clients are very hazy about words which become another defense. But if you do a dance that feels like love, a dance that feels like looking for one's center --not trying to find a word for that--the word will come, after true experience in the delving. There is an analogy between the meaningful word and meaningful dance improvisation. I developed ways of initiating creative improvisation for the purpose of stripping styles and habits from movement. Fresh movement evolves. Its content is that of the clients' and trainees' therapy problems. Improvisation as I use it exists when the person has given all of herself to its power. It deals in memory and psychophysical associations. Honest improvisation in dance is a direct route to the unconscious. Training includes studying improvisation which uses creative dance as its base while constantly enriching it through concentration, depth, and an increase of movement vocabulary.

I: In closing, then, would you summarize your objectives in dance therapy with your clients? It's a huge question.

Blanche: Haven't I answered that yet?

I: Yes you have, but if you would pull it together in your own way...

Blanche: To grow, from confusion to clarity to practice. To develop the strength to make the statement. To arrive at self-choice of one's identity: sexual, social, economic, whatever. The growth that leads the client towards eventual self-therapy. For the client to build her courage in transforming insight into action and renewing the sense of the totality of her person. To continue to challenge the narcissism of our American culture, not to revert to the solitude of the secret, but to keep breaking down the secret.

I: After listening to your responses, I am reminded that you always had a great personal and often poetic way of using words.

Blanche: Thank you, Iris. Last night I went through my little notebook where I write spontaneous thoughts that come to me. Here are a few: "In my work the objective is in the method. Objective and method are one.

"Reality in a neurotic world is that for which no fantasies can be found."

"We don't 'feel', we work"

"You become greater, not by being someone else, but by being unflinchingly more yourself."

"When in doubt, study."

"A neurotic is in his own trap, or prison, or playpen, spends a lot of time (the lost years) pretending he wants to get out."

"When crying is a block, it equates with self pity."

"What seems spontaneous, is that moment of a chain reaction...often it is the missing link."

But I also know the other side of the world where, despite our efforts, I know how alone we are, how lonely we are and how we hold on to what we believe in, despite lack of encouragement or understanding.

I was walking down the street in Carmel where there are pretty gardens of flowers and I saw them and sat down and this is what I wrote:

Poem

A million fields of flowers

      Before I die to see

       them, every kind and variety

      Tall touching the sun

       (or so they believe)

      short stemmed cuddled

by the earth

      wide petalled to

       east and west, like

       the horizon with

       no beginning and no

       end--

On death row the prisoner

      is asked..one last request?

      " field of flowers, mostly

pink and purple, wide and

       high and forever"

      "I told you she was crazy, "the

       executioner whispered

      as he pressed the switch, pulled the

      rope, or fired the last shot

I: (There was a deep silence. We clasped hands and said a silent good night.)

"Reprinted by permission from American Journal of Dance Therapy, Volume V, 1982"

Unpublished Works
By Blanche Evan

Functional Technique

with drawings by Mary Loomis Wilson

The Dance - Modernistic...Whither?

An American at The Soviet Union Ballet

Rejection Has Many Faces

The Body Language A Road to Reality

The Modern Dance, An Analysis for Teachers and Students

The Teaching of Rhythmic Dancing

Creative Dancing in America - "In My Red Tunic"

Other Resources

Levy, Fran J., "Blanche Evan: Creative Movement Becomes Dance Therapy With Normals and Neurotics," in DANCE MOVEMENT THERAPY A HEALING ART, The American Alliance for Health, Physical Education, Recreation, and Dance, Reston, Va., 1988, pp. 33-49.

Rifkin-Gainer, I., Bernstein, B., Melson, B., "Dance/Movement/Word Therapy: The Methods of Blanche Evan," in Bernstein, P., THEORETICAL APPROACHES IN DANCE-MOVEMENT THERAPY VOL. II, Kendall/Hunt Publishing, Dubuque, Iowa, 1988, pp. 3-62.

Melson, Barbara, "Body Image and Its Relation to Self Concept in Individual Dance Therapy Sessions with a Normal Adult Male," Unpublished Masters Thesis, Hunter College, 1980.

Personal Communication

It is not possible to publish the vast amount of letters received by Blanche Evan from students, dancers, schools, psychologists, psychiatrists, artists, etc. The following is a small sample of the thousands she received over the span of her professional life.

copy of the communication.

Ruth St. Denis   *3433 Cahuenga Blvd.*   *Hollywood, California*   *HI 9892*

Columbia University
in the City of New York

DEPARTMENT OF MUSIC

Monday
March 23/36

Dear Blanche Evan:

Just a word to tell you how
profoundly moved I was by your dance
"In Meekness" last night.   It
portrayed with rare and subtle insight
the character of a person who lives
in the shadow world of his own
timidity. All the little weaknesses,
the timid venturings forth, the sometimes
bravura acting that with a fine play
raises the person to the level of a
free,brave man: the hidden spectres
looming ghostlike in his soul, the dream-
phantasy, the unreal world in which he
lives - are all given out in the strange,
haunting quality of the dance.

It is as deep and penetrating
as a psychological study, but more alive
and virile, translated from the inner
consciousness into clear, lucid
movement. Always at the moment when it
retains its most phantom-like quality,
it is most real and easily understandable.

By the very strength of its
conception, it pierces the hidden
pitiable weaknesses of a creature of
timid aspirations, small horizons, weak
and frail convictions. And like a
drifting leaf it is borne along on every
wind, every current that uproots it
from its insecure and slender base.

The play of the hands,
the delicate summoning of pretense, the
strange acting are all part of the picture
you draw to uncannily lifelike proportions.

I have never seen anything
like it and was thrilled and excited,
and wanted you to know about it.

Sincerely,

Florence Ungar

PEPI MILLER, PH. D.
PSYCHOLOGIST

349 EAST 49TH STREET
NEW YORK 17
ELDORADO 5-1770

April 9, 1962

To Whom It May Concern:

Miss Blanche Evan has for the past three years been
assisting me as an auxilliary therapist and I have found
her sufficiently unique to be distinctive in her ability
to handle children as well as adults in dance therapy and
rehabilitation.

There is a sincerity and dedication in Miss Evan's work
with her patients that is indeed rare.

Sincerely,

Pepi Miller

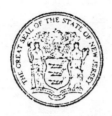

State of New Jersey

MONTCLAIR STATE COLLEGE

AT MONTCLAIR

August 1, 1962

Dear Miss Evan:

In December of 1959 you were kind enough to give me the benefit of your knowledge in contributing to a study undertaken at New York University concerning the principle of opposition as related to movement in dance. Your comments were most helpful, and assisted greatly in the realization of the study. It is now on file under the title, The Nature of Opposition, in the library of New York University. A quotation of your statement appears within pages 53--56.

Sincerely,

Patricia Sparrow
Assistant Professor of
Dance and Physical Education

1938

Blanche my darling —

We talked at least a year ago on what the dance might do for artists. Well, it's doing that, and more for me. It's making me more alive and expressive and better aware of the body, the structure, the loveliness of its movements. It's such an unexpected joy to me, the way it keeps coming into my mind.

Now I'm planning 4 bigger (than before) paintings on 4 related subjects and I assure you, the dance will be in them though it can't be seen.

Mary

Mary Wilson is the artist who drew all the dance and body sketches for Blanche Evan's book, FUNCTIONAL TECHNIQUE.

IIP

INSTITUTE FOR INDIVIDUAL PSYCHOLOGY

333 CENTRAL PARK WEST   NEW YORK 25, N. Y.   MOnument 3-7980

February 1958

Director:
Helene Papanek, M.D.

Co-Director:
Alfred Farau, Ph.D.

TO WHOM IT MAY CONCERN :

This is to certify that

Miss BLANCHE EVAN

has successfully completed a two-year course
in Adlerian Psychology at our Institute for
Individual Psychology, New York, N.Y., begun
in October 1955 and terminated in June 1957.
At the end of   submitted an able
paper: " Life as Movement."

       Evan, who has met all the requirements
of the Institute, is at present taking some additional courses with us. She is held in high regard
by the faculty.

Helene Papanek M D

Heléne Papanek, M.D.,
Director

Alfred Farau, Ph. D.

Alfred Farau, Ph.D.,
Co-Director

DANCE REVIEWS

"One of the best "An office Girl Dreams" which blended humor and wistfulness and had the further advantage of excellent and eclinecal achievement."

> Herald Tribune
> Jerome D. Bohm

"Mme. Evan revela un rare dynamisme artistique, facilement divers, mais toujours profond.   Elle temo gne une technique minutieuse, avertie, intellectuelle."

> Montreal La Presse

"... possesses a fine sense of what the art of the dance really stands for ... muscular control impeccable ... skilled and subtle choreography ... a dancer to be reckoned with ... safe to prophesy a brilliant future for this gifted young dancer ..."

> Montreal Gazette
> Thomas Archer

"A young artist of uncommon promise. She is graceful and lithe and has a living sense of rhythm. The muscular control was impeccable in "Demand"...not to mention the utterly charming "Contre Tanz", the performance of which alone stamps Miss Evan as a dancer to be reckoned with."

> Montreal Gazette

"... brings to her audience ... perception of the principal forces at work in the contemporary scene ...."

> New Masses

"Blanche Evan appeared on the program in a strong and challenging light. The suite had clear conception and directness. Miss Evan revealed an objectivity of approach which, for the young dancers, has always been one of the most difficult things to maintain."

> New Theatre Magazine, New York

"... able to project her idea through symbology ... pantomine ... movement. 'Slum Child' even more moving ... heart-felt ... heart breaking ...."

> Boston Christian Science Monitor
> Margaret Lloyd

"... She has a richness of gesture and a wealth of feeling that she transmits to her audience ... a moving rhythm and a remarkable musical understanding ..."

> New York Post

"... imagination and versatility ... and innate sense of satire ... original style ... poignant portrayal ...."

> American Dancer
> Frederick L. Orme

"... clean incisive movements ... excellent control ... dances with authority and the assurance that comes of ability ...."

> Dance Magazine
> Joseph Arnold Kaye

".....Miss Evan's original interpretations were always interesting. Physically, she is the most competent dancer that we have had here since Pavlova--which goes back some fifteen years. She uses none of the conventional arts of the ballerina. Her work is of the purely objective character of which Mary Wigman is today the principle exponent. And, like Fraulein Wigman, she has that alert intelligence and fluidity of muscle which combine to make a vibrant, resilient and often beautiful performance. Her costumes, also of original design, were colorful and in excellent taste....."

> WHEELING NEWS-REGISTER,
> West Virginia, Robert Permar

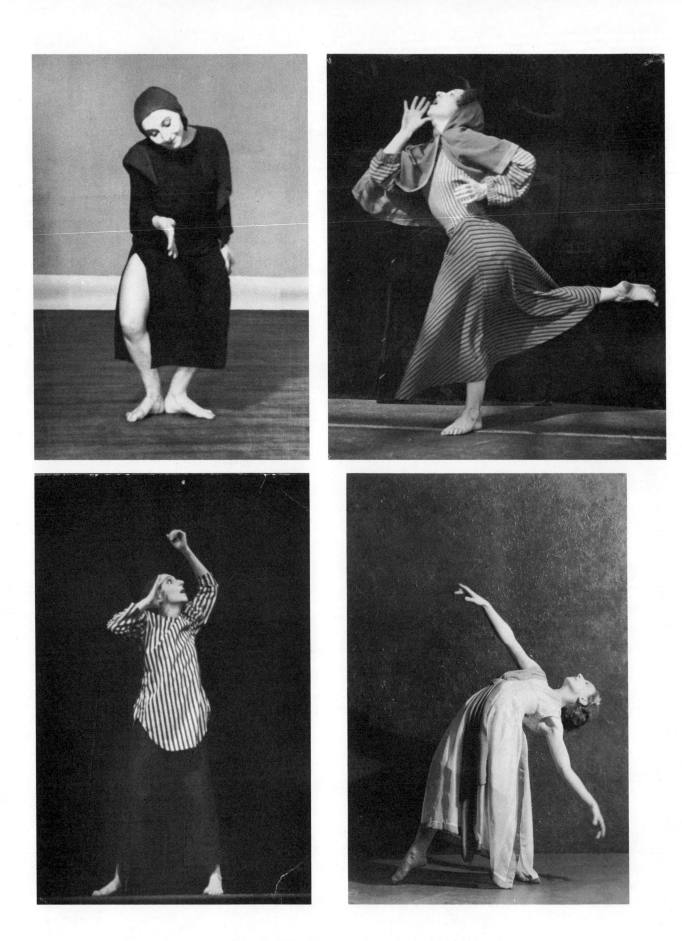

Solo Concert, Labor Stage Theater, New York City

Collected Works By and About Blanche Evan

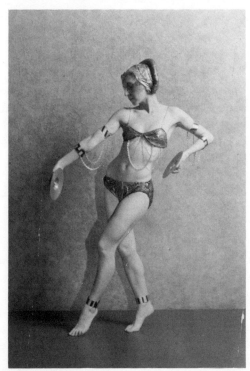

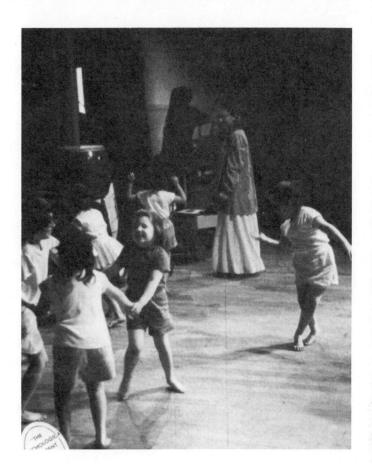

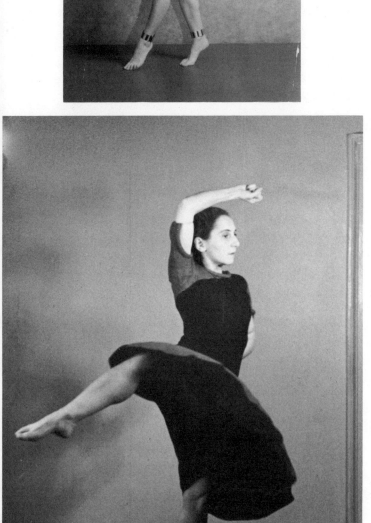

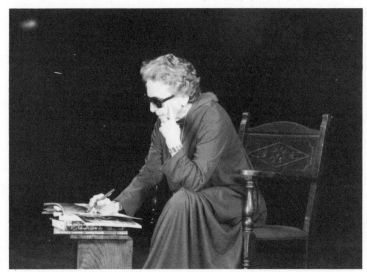

As a young dancer, concert performer, teacher and writer/therapist.

Ruth Gordon Benov

We met at the Roerich Museum in New York City sometime around 1931. Blanche Evan was teaching a class in adult creative dance. I enrolled and stayed with Blanche till her death in December 1982--first as a student, then as a member of her dance company, later as her manager and, always, her friend.

Ruth Gordon Benov taught creative dance to children and adults for 30 years in her own studio in Queens, New York. The school held a special division for children with impaired hearing, cerebral palsy, mental retardation and minimal brain dysfunction. In addition, Mrs. Benov held a position as dance therapist in New York City elementary schools and Queens General Hospital. She holds certification in "AIM" (Adventures in Movement for the Handicapped), as well as a certificate from the Dance Therapy Centre in New York City. Mrs. Benov has taught a graduate course in movement and kinetic awareness at C.W. Post College.

More recently, Mrs. Benov held a position as dance therapist at The Lorge School in New York City, where she worked with children with various emotional and learning problems. She achieved the position of Administrative Director at that school and retired from the position in 1986.

Ruth Gordon Benov currently lives in New York City.

Bonnie Bernstein

Bonnie Bernstein began intensive study with Blanche Evan at age 18. She was a college student seeking to bridge her lifelong love of dance with an increasing interest in psychology. Experiencing an immediate resonance with the person and her work, she entered into thirteen years of intensive study and training with Blanche Evan.

Bonnie graduated from Goddard College, with a major in Dance Therapy based on a three year apprenticeship with Blanche Evan. After graduation, she joined the staff at The Dance Therapy Centre, leading groups and individual sessions and assisting Blanche in training courses. Until Blanche's death, she remained Bonnie's mentor, supervisor, teacher, therapist and friend. This multifaceted relationship facilitated invaluable insights into Blanche's techniques and her philosophy of Dance, Movement, Word Therapy.

Bonnie completed a Masters in Counseling at Boston University and received certification as an ADTR. In the area of dance ethnology, she has traveled to research the therapeutic use of dance in West Africa and Malaysia. Working with individuals and groups she has maintained her own dance therapy practice since 1975. As a consultant for the City of New York she led dance therapy groups for older adults for over 11 years. From 1978-1984 she was an adjunct professor at Long Island University, C.W.Post Center.

After moving to California in 1983, Bonnie became a licensed Marriage, Family and Child Counselor. She developed a dance therapy program at a multidisciplinary physical rehabilitation clinic in San Francisco. In the past eight years she has specialized in therapy for survivors of sexual assault. This has included training of volunteers working with this population. Bonnie has led dance therapy workshops both in the U.S. and abroad.

Throughout her twenty years of training and work as a therapist, the essence of Bonnie's work has always remained Dance Therapy, in the methods of Blanche Evan. Her foundation in the Blanche Evan approach to therapy remains a wellspring of her creativity as a therapist.

She currently has a private practice and works with the Palo Alto Rape Crisis Center.

Bonnie lives with her husband, daughter and son in Palo Alto, California.

Anne Krantz

Nearly twenty years after my first meeting with Blanche Evan, my first impressions are clear. Physically, she was a commanding presence, authoritative and artistic. I attended a presentation of dances created by her students and clients. As a dancer myself, I saw for the first time, dances expressing very personal and very powerful feelings. The effect on me was profound, evoking and opening my own feelings. This was the kind of dance I wanted to do; it had the honesty and depth I searched for in my own improvisations.

Blanche's uncanny way of targeting the psychophysical issues in her clients was a unique skill which we, her trainees, were always seeking to learn. We would ask,"can you teach perception, or how you use your life experience, or how to distill ideas into action, or stir stagnation into change?" "You cannot be me" she would tell us, always challenging us to use our own creativity, perception, skills, and experience in work with our clients. Blanche Evan's methods can be experienced, taught and read about. Painstakingly developed in fifty years of work with children and adults, they exist now in the work of those who continued training with her and who practice today. We have been given the tools, "like a plumber" Blanche would say, of her system of therapy, technique, and creative dance.

The person Blanche Evan is gone, more than eight years to this date. Understanding her complex personality illuminates the body of work she created. Her often enigmatic qualities made her an object both loved and emulated by colleagues, students, and friends. Uncompromising regarding her beliefs, ideals and life view, she was driven time and time again to stand as an individual alone against institutions and conventions which deaden, numb, and disempower people. Blanche was a genius in her creative realm, an iconoclast, artist, activist, and foremost, a teacher. Her whole being went into her work. She engaged with her clients and students intimately, passionately, and with respect, believing completely in their potential and in their basic right to be whole, free human beings.

Working with individual clients or leading large groups, Blanche embodied what was needed to guide them, to draw them out, to model honesty, concentration, and work, and to support their confrontations with problems and potential for change. She had the gift to inspire others to reach their own depths and heights. As she worked, the magnificent power of creativity to heal was manifested and was taught to her clients, as they transmuted stagnant emotion into meaningful action. The outcome was self-empowerment and the objective, a better way of life. As she wrote, "first, the human being, second, a better person toward a better world." A pragmatic individualist with socially cooperative ideals, Blanche understood that enlarging and interconnecting systems, beginning with the self, was the ultimate goal. With Blanche, there was never a question of honesty. She did as she was.

Anne Krantz worked with Blanche Evan from 1973 until her death in 1982, becoming a dance therapist and teacher under her training and supervision. Also a choreographer and dancer, Anne performed solo concerts from 1976-84 in Northern California, Colorado, New York, Washington, Europe and India. Her repertory included "FLOOR/FLIGHT/FEET", choreographed by Blanche Evan in 1981. From 1984-1988 she performed with the Brynar Mehl Dance Company in San Francisco. Her dedication to the practice of both dance and dance therapy has been a guiding force in her professional development. Since 1976 she has been in private practice as a dance therapist and teaching creative dance based in Blanche Evan methods. Her work with adults, adolescents, and children has included clients with physical and learning disabilities, eating disorders, and survivors of sexual abuse. Formerly on the faculty of Santa Rosa Junior College, Anne has given workshops and classes at colleges and institutes, including Sonoma State University, Antioch College, Sonoma Institute, and the Movement Therapy Institute, Seattle. Anne is currently working toward a doctorate in Clinical Psychology and maintains her ongoing commitment to Evan's teachings and methods.

Anne lives in San Francisco with her husband and two daughters.

Barbara Melson

Barbara Melson was introduced to dance at the age of four when she began classes in Creative Dance with Ruth Gordon Benov. She studied with Ms. Benov until the age of nine. At sixteen, she resumed the study of dance and began to study Modern Dance. After receiving a B.A. in Dance from the University of Colorado in 1973, she moved to New York City to study with Blanche Evan. At that time, she discovered that Ms. Evan and Ms. Benov were colleagues and friends and that her childhood creative dance experiences had laid the foundation for her work with Blanche Evan's dance therapy.

As Barbara began to study intensively with Blanche Evan, she felt a tremendous affinity with her beliefs and methods. She continued to study with her from 1973 until Ms. Evan's death in 1982. At various stages in this relationship Ms. Evan was teacher, therapist, mentor and friend. She had a profound impact on Barbara's personal and professional life and remains the primary influence in her work.

Barbara has worked as a dance therapist and creative dance teacher in the New York area for the past fifteen years. In the mid to late seventies she was on the staff of the Blanche Evan Dance Therapy Centre. In addition, she worked for the Cultural Enrichment Program of the New York City Department of Parks and Recreation--in community day programs for geriatrics--and taught creative dance to children in day care settings. She has also worked as a dance therapist with adolescent and adult psychiatric patients and substance abusers at Gracie Square Hospital in New York City and Fair Oaks Hospital in Summit, New Jersey. She is a member of the Academy of Registered Dance Therapists.

Barbara has an M.S. in dance therapy from Hunter College and has been a guest lecturer and supervisor in that program. Following completion of her masters degree, she integrated models of group dance therapy and group psychotherapy with Blanche Evan's methods and used this integrative model in work with psychiatric patients in day treatment and in-patient settings.

In private practice in New York City since 1975, Ms. Melson's work in depth dance psychotherapy is based in the methods of Blanche Evan. She has led and co-led training and experiential workshops in Blanche Evan methods, has taught creative dance to adults, and provided supervision to therapists and students. Her private work is primarily with women and often focuses on body image issues and related concerns.

Barbara currently lives in Brooklyn Heights, New York with her husband and two daughters.

Iris Rifkin-Gainer

Iris Rifkin-Gainer first came to the studio in 1947, at the age of three, to study Creative Dance with Blanche Evan. She continued to work with her until her death in 1982, as the work evolved from Creative Dance to Dance Therapy. During Miss Evan's one year absence from New York, Iris was Director of The Blanche Evan Dance Therapy Centre.

She was Adjunct Assistant Professor on the faculty of New York University's Graduate Dance Therapy Program from 1970-1985 and has been a guest teacher at Smith College, Naropa Institute, Bucknell University and Roehampton College, London. She has also taught Creative Dance to children and had a Dance Therapy practice with adults, utilizing Blanche Evan's methods in N.Y.C. and Connecticut and has given workshops in the methods in N.Y.C., Ct., Boulder and London. Among these workshops which are committed to both the Creative Dance work and Dance Therapy methods of Blanche Evan, are those co-led with Barbara Melson. Iris has also participated in a jointly led professional presentation with Barbara Melson, Anne Krantz and Bonnie Bernstein in the same vein. She has published on Miss Evan's work.

Iris currently resides in Lewisburg, Pennsylvania with her husband and daughter.

ACKNOWLEDGEMENTS

The Blanche Evan Dance Foundation wishes to thank the people listed below who helped make this publication possible, as well as those contributors whose gifts arrived after the book had gone to press.

ざ   ざ   ざ   ざ

Maja Apelman; Pamela Armel; Judith Bell; Ruth Gordon Benov; Bonnie, Daniel, Alissa and Adam Bernstein; Freda Birnbaum; Ellen and Gerson Bodner; Harriet Bograd; Geraldine M. Burke; Susan A. Campodonico; Sharon Chaiklin; Marsha and Jerry Connell; Bonnie B. Benov Danus and Richard Danus; Kira C. Danus; D'Arcy Masius Benton & Bowles; Wendy Dreskin; Peggy Drexler; Mrs. Bert Druck; Judi and Michael Druck; Charles Evan; In memory of Dora Weiszner Friedman; Iris Rifkin-Gainer; Andrea Gitter; Marcelle Grant; The Gunther Family; Beth Ann Handler; Dassie Hoffman; Sandra Indig; Miriam and Mark Jacoby; Michael Kidd; The Kirschenbaum and Cantor Family; Berti Klein; Nancy Koprak; Beth Krackov, Anne Krantz and Mark Gunther; Lois La Fond and Family; Jane Lazar; Shoshanna Lederman; Dr. Marcia B. Leventhal; Joan L. (Naess) Lewin; Jeannette List; Jane Margules; Laura McDonnell; Carol Evan McKeand and Nigel McKeand; Duncan Meaney; Barbara Melson and Joseph Ganz; Mr. and Mrs. Harold W. Melson; Clare Venet Meltzer; Margot Mink; Pat Mowry; Dr. Nurit R. Mussen; Ragnar D. Naess; Carol and Richard Nathan; Linda S. Newman; John and Pat O'Neil; Gayle Reid; Clifford and Monica Rosenberg; Zalman Rosenfeld; Claire Schmais; Georgette Schneer; Alice and Michael Schure; Mady Schutzman; Dr. Stephan Sheppard; Anne Herbert Smith; Barbara Somerfield; Benita Somerfield; Joseph and Muriel Spanier; Nancy Spanier; Tamara Spolan; Adrienne Fabrizio-Todd; Sunday K. Tyner; Janet Wice; Ruth Winneck.

PUBLICATIONS
AVAILABLE FROM
THE BLANCHE EVAN
DANCE FOUNDATION

Blanche Evan Dance Foundation is dedicated to publishing and promoting the work of Blanche Evan.

Currently available from the foundation are:

Collected Works By And About Blanche Evan
Published 1991 $34.95

Please inquire for Reseller discount.

Reprint: A Series of Articles by Blanche Evan.

The Child's World and It's Relation to Dance Pedagogy
Reprinted from Dance Magazine 1949-1951 $15.00

A Packet of Pieces by and About Blanche Evan
Published and Unpublished Work 1945-1978 $15.00

Please Order From:

**Blanche Evan Dance Foundation
c/o Anne Krantz
146 5th Avenue
San Francisco, California 94118
(415) 387-0621**

With Special Thanks......

To all former dance and dance therapy students of Blanche Evan who are now practicing and teaching in France, Israel, Colorado, Arizona, California and New York City.

To Esther Klein Friedman - For sensitive editorial advice.

To Ivette Torres Ortiz - For her thorough secretarial services.

To Bonnie Bernstein, Anne Krantz, Barbara Melson, Iris Rifkin-Gainer -

I give my everlasting gratitude for their devotion and the continuation of the Blanche Evan Methods.

To Carol Evan McKeand I say -

Without your trust and love, this book could not have been.

To Blanche -

"Hearing you praised I say, `Tis so, `tis true; and to the most of the praise add something more." (Shakespeare)

Ruth Gordon Benov